A Practical Guide to Heart Failure in Older People

A Practical Guide to Heart Failure in Older People

Editors

Christopher Ward
and
Miles D. Witham
Ninewells Hospital, Dundee, UK

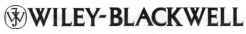

WILEY-BLACKWELL

A John Wiley & Sons, Ltd., Publication

This edition first published 2009
© 2009 John Wiley & Sons, Ltd

Wiley-Blackwell is an imprint of John Wiley & Sons, formed by the merger of Wiley's global Scientific, Technical and Medical business with Blackwell Publishing.

Registered office: John Wiley & Sons Ltd, The Atrium, Southern Gate, Chichester, West Sussex, PO19 8SQ, UK

Other Editorial Offices:
9600 Garsington Road, Oxford, OX4 2DQ, UK
111 River Street, Hoboken, NJ 07030-5774, USA

For details of our global editorial offices, for customer services and for information about how to apply for permission to reuse the copyright material in this book please see our website at www.wiley.com/wiley-blackwell

The right of the author to be identified as the author of this work has been asserted in accordance with the Copyright, Designs and Patents Act 1988.

Wiley also publishes its books in a variety of electronic formats. Some content that appears in print may not be available in electronic books.

Designations used by companies to distinguish their products are often claimed as trademarks. All brand names and product names used in this book are trade names, service marks, trademarks or registered trademarks of their respective owners. The publisher is not associated with any product or vendor mentioned in this book. This publication is designed to provide accurate and authoritative information in regard to the subject matter covered. It is sold on the understanding that the publisher is not engaged in rendering professional services. If professional advice or other expert assistance is required, the services of a competent professional should be sought.

The contents of this work are intended to further general scientific research, understanding, and discussion only and are not intended and should not be relied upon as recommending or promoting a specific method, diagnosis, or treatment by physicians for any particular patient. The publisher and the author make no representations or warranties with respect to the accuracy or completeness of the contents of this work and specifically disclaim all warranties, including without limitation any implied warranties of fitness for a particular purpose. In view of ongoing research, equipment modifications, changes in governmental regulations, and the constant flow of information relating to the use of medicines, equipment, and devices, the reader is urged to review and evaluate the information provided in the package insert or instructions for each medicine, equipment, or device for, among other things, any changes in the instructions or indication of usage and for added warnings and precautions. Readers should consult with a specialist where appropriate. The fact that an organization or Website is referred to in this work as a citation and/or a potential source of further information does not mean that the author or the publisher endorses the information the organization or Website may provide or recommendations it may make. Further, readers should be aware that Internet Websites listed in this work may have changed or disappeared between when this work was written and when it is read. No warranty may be created or extended by any promotional statements for this work. Neither the publisher nor the author shall be liable for any damages arising herefrom.

Library of Congress Cataloguing-in-Publication Data

A practical guide to heart failure in older people/[edited by]
Christopher Ward, Miles Witham.
     p. ; cm.
  Includes bibliographical references and index.
  ISBN 978-0-470-69517-3 (cloth)
 1. Heart failure. 2. Geriatric cardiology. I. Ward, Christopher,
1939- II. Witham, Miles.
  [DNLM: 1. Heart Failure–therapy. 2. Aged. WG 370 P8955 2009]
  RC685.C53P733 2009
  618.97'129–dc22   2009004190

ISBN: 978-0-470-69517-3 (H/B)

A catalogue record for this book is available from the British Library.

Typeset in 10.5/13pt Minion by Thomson Digital, Noida, India.
Printed in Great Britain by CPI Antony Rowe, Chippenham, Wiltshire
[First impression   2009]

Contents

Preface

Numerous books have been written about heart failure, and both international and local treatment guidelines are readily available. But the information they contain about heart failure in older people is limited: It has to be identified piecemeal - from brief accounts in book chapters, which are usually limited in scope or, for more detailed information on specific topics, from articles in journals.

The lack of trial evidence advocating the use of standard "heart failure medicines" in older people (and their consequent sub optimal treatment) is well known, but this doesn't apply to most other age-related topics. These include epidemiological predictions that the prevalence of heart failure in older patients (currently 10% in the over 80s) is set to increase dramatically in the next few decades with major implications for healthcare provision; the complex interaction of common comorbidities with heart failure in older patients which hampers diagnosis and adversely affects disease progression and treatment; and research into the normal aging of the cardiovascular system, much of it during the past 10 years or so, which has a dramatic effect on the prevalence, aetiology, gender differences and prognosis of heart failure. And whereas summarising the treatment of heart failure (i.e. the appropriate pharmacological, non pharmacological and interventional options) is relatively straightforward, the same cannot be said of patient management (i.e. how best to provided treatment and care): it is more complicated and time consuming in those who are older as they are often frail and socially isolated . As a result they are more dependent on medical and nursing support and on input from social services.

Based on these observations, a good case can be made for regarding heart failure in older and younger patients, certainly in a number of respects, as different diseases.

Our aim has been to present heart failure in much the same format as it is in other books on the subject but here the subject matter is focused on how the disease impacts on older patients and their personal carers, and on the health care teams (in primary care and secondary care teams and specialist heart failure nurses) whose responsibility it is to identify and treat, and to collaborate in caring for them.

Acknowledgements

We are grateful to Dr Derek MacLean for his contributions to the editing process and for his wise advice and support during the preparation of this book; to Professor Hugh Tunstall-Pedoe for invaluable advice on the writing of chapter 2; and to Teresa Coppinger, sister in charge of the Heart Failure Clinic at South Manchester University Hospital NHS Trust: Many years ago she encouraged and gently cajoled CW, then a recently appointed cardiologist, to develop a special interest in heart failure and to help her to establish a heart failure clinic there (probably the first such clinic in the UK) in the mid 1980s. Without her encouragement to develop that interest, this book would not have been written.

C Ward

List of Contributors

Alan G. Begg

General Practitioner
Hon Senior Lecturer
University of Dundee
Townhead Practice
Links Health Centre
Montrose
DD10 8TY, UK

Francis G. Dunn

Consultant Cardiologist
Cardiac Department
Stobhill Hospital
Glasgow
G21 3UW, UK

Andrew Elder

Consultant in Acute Elderly Medicine
Honorary Senior Lecturer
Anne Ferguson Building
Western General Hospital
Crewe Road
Edinburgh
EH4 2XU, UK

Andrew Hannah

Consultant cardiologist
Department of Cardiology
Aberdeen Royal Infirmary
Foresterhill
Aberdeen
AB25 2ZN, UK

Shona M. M. Jenkins

Research Fellow
Cardiac Department
Stobhill Hospital
Glasgow
G21 3UW, UK

Chim C. Lang

Professor of Cardiology
Division of Medicine and
Therapeutics
University of Dundee
Ninewells Hospital and Medical
School
Dundee
DD1 9SY, UK

J. Martin Leiper

Consultant in Palliative Medicine
NHS Tayside
UK

Stephen J. Leslie

Consultant Cardiologist
and Honorary Reader
Highland Heartbeat Centre
Cardiac Unit
Raigmore Hospital
Inverness
IV2 3UJ, UK

Sinéad P. McKee

Cardiology Specialist Nurse
Cardiac Rehabilitation Team
Stirling Royal Infirmary
Livilands Gate
Stirling
FK8 2AU, UK

Helen Oxenham

Consultant Cardiologist
Cardiology Department
Borders General Hospital
Melrose
Roxburghshire
TD6 9BS, UK

Maheshwar Pauriah

TMRC Research Fellow
Division of Medicine and
Therapeutics
University of Dundee
Ninewells Hospital and
Medical School
Dundee
DD1 9SY, UK

Christopher Ward

Honorary Consultant Cardiologist
Ninewells Hospital and Medical School
Dundee
DD1 9SY, UK
Contact address
2 Hazel Gardens
Dundee, Scotland
DD2 1UF, UK
chrisav@btopenworld.com

Martin Wilson

Consultant Physician
Care of the Elderly
Raigmore Hospital
Inverness
IV2 3UJ, UK

Miles D. Witham

Clinician Scientist in Ageing and Health
Section of Ageing and Health
Ninewells Hospital
Dundee
DD1 9SY, UK

Aaron Wong

BHF Research Fellow
Division of Medicine and Therapeutics
University of Dundee
Ninewells Hospital and Medical School
Dundee
DD1 9SY, UK

1

Introduction

Christopher Ward

Ninewells Hospital and Medical School, Dundee

Key messages

- The problems associated with treating heart failure in older patients are more diverse and complex than in those who are younger.

- The paucity of evidence-based guidelines for treating older patients results in many having suboptimal management.

- The expectations of older and younger patients are broadly similar.

1.1 A working definition of heart failure (see also Chapter 5)

There have been numerous attempts to define heart failure. Some are convoluted and others barely intelligible or else impractical [1]: none has been generally approved. This situation has arisen for two reasons. First, the underlying defect in all cases of heart failure – the inability of the left ventricle to eject sufficient blood to meet the body's metabolic needs – is not exclusively caused by myocardial damage; it can result from diseases of the pericardium, endocardium or great vessels [2], and a concise definition to incorporate all of these pathologies is elusive. Second, there is no general agreement about what, in objective terms, constitutes left ventricular impairment.

A Practical Guide to Heart Failure in Older People, Edited by C Ward and M D Witham
© 2009 John Wiley & Sons, Ltd

The European Society of Cardiology: Guidelines for the Diagnosis and Treatment of Chronic Heart Failure [3] have taken a pragmatic approach to this by identifying the essential components of the syndrome of heart failure as follows:

- Symptoms of heart failure, typically breathlessness or fatigue at rest or on exertion or ankle swelling, plus

- Objective evidence of left ventricular dysfunction at rest: this is usually obtained by means of echocardiography.

The American Heart Association guidelines [2] define heart failure in broadly similar terms.

This is clearly not a definition in the conventional sense of the word; it is a précis of the diagnostic criteria.

The Scottish Intercollegiate Network Guideline SIGN 95 [4] has, however, provided a succinct, but unavoidably imprecise definition:

> "Chronic heart failure is a complex clinical syndrome that can result from any structural or functional cardiac or non cardiac disorder that impairs the ability of the heart to respond to physiological demands for increased cardiac output."

1.2   What do we mean by 'older people?'

There are many occasions in medical and legal practice, and in the provision of public services, when there is a need to know an individual's age. Although such specific information is unnecessary in the context of this book, it is important to identify in broader terms the age group of the patients we will be discussing and to understand why it has been chosen.

In the US and the UK the word 'elderly' usually refers to people of retirement age and above, as does the ubiquitous use of the phrase 'heart failure in the elderly' in the medical press. But many current 65- and 70-year-old people, quite rightly, do not regard themselves as 'elderly' (the meaning of which is explained in vague terms as 'somewhat old; past middle age' [5]), although logically they would accept that they are 'older'. We will therefore use this term in place of 'elderly' with all of its negative connotations.

When an age limit is set for a particular purpose or action, it usually implies that adults who are above that age: (i) may be unable to safely engage in the activity in question; (ii) that existing rules or regulations cannot or should no longer apply to them; or (iii) they are of an age when additional medical, financial or social support may be needed. By and large, in the United Kingdom these statements are applied to those who have reached the current State pension age. This is therefore the age at which it is generally accepted or assumed that a wide range of biological changes begin to occur.

There are arguments both for and against using this as the age at which we might be called 'older'.

Epidemiological and social data suggest that many 65-year-olds are biologically, socially and functionally younger than this:

- We now live considerably longer than when the first contributory pension scheme was introduced in the UK in 1925. At that time, the average male life expectancy beyond the age of 65 was approximately 4 years, whereas now it is more than 15 years [6].

- Increasing numbers of people remain in employment and/or regularly engage in physically and intellectually demanding activities well beyond the traditional retirement age.

- In the medical context, the older people become, the more heterogeneous they become physiologically and functionally. It is now recognized that with respect to survival, biological age is more important than chronological age [7].

However, not everybody over the age of 65 is biologically young, and our objectives in writing this book are to highlight and to address the numerous important differences between younger and older patients with heart failure.

- The pathological changes, and the normal aging processes which are responsible for these differences are initiated well before the current retirement age, and it is in the seventh decade of life that their impact in causing an escalation in the prevalence of heart failure becomes evident.

- Most clinical trials on which the management of heart failure is based effectively excluded patients beyond their mid sixties. As a result, most information on which diagnosis, treatment and management are based is skewed towards the 20% of the heart failure population aged under the age of 65.

- We are surviving and remaining active and healthy for longer, but epidemiological reports show that we also spend longer in poor health. In fact, the prediction is that heart failure in older people will become more – not less – prevalent during the coming decades (see Chapter 2).

Consequently, because of the epidemiological data and our objectives, and despite the evidence that many of us are 'getting younger', we made a pragmatic decision to accept what is in effect the existing widely accepted 'definition' of elderly: we will use 'older' to describe patients above the age of about 65–70 years.

1.3   The expectations of older patients

In general terms, the natural history of heart failure is the same irrespective of age; a symptomatic improvement in response to treatment, a period of stability and, after a variable time, progressive deterioration often punctuated by periods of decompensation resulting in hospitalization; during this period, up to 50% of patients die suddenly and unexpectedly.

Most older patients want the same outcomes from their treatment as do younger patients – symptom relief, a better quality of life and an improved prognosis. The optimum means of achieving these objectives are also the same: guideline-based medication (although most of the medicines were evaluated in younger patients), plus surgery, interventional treatments and palliative and supportive care when appropriate.

However, when patients are old and frail they may regard treatment which offers an improvement in the quality of their remaining life as being preferable to increased longevity, especially as they may have comorbidities which are more distressing than their heart failure. Consequently, they may prefer more conservative care, whereas a biologically young older patient may wish, and is entitled, to be considered for the same surgical or interventional treatments offered to younger patients (see Chapter 10).

1.4   Age-related problems in heart failure treatment and management

Although the principles of treatment and management are independent of age, the similarities between the care of younger and older patients effectively end there. The problems faced by older patients, their families and friends, and by the health care teams caring for them, are more diverse and complex than those of younger patients. They affect all aspects of treatment and management and have important implications for the strategic planning of future services (Table 1.1).

The effective management of older patients requires a clear understanding of each of these problems, of how they differ from those in younger patients, and of how best they can be addressed:

- Heart failure is more common, and the prognosis worse, in older patients.

- The prevalence of heart failure is increasing, and will continue to do so as life expectancy – and specifically survival from myocardial infarction – continue to improve.

- Significant anatomical, physiological and biochemical changes occur in the cardiovascular system with aging. These age-related changes are responsible for

Table 1.1 Age-related differences between older and younger patients with heart failure which affect diagnosis, management and treatment.

Parameter	Young/middle-aged	Older
Prevalence	1–2%	8–10%[a]
Incidence	2/1000	30/1000[a]
Prognosis	Bad	Worse[a]
Left ventricular systolic function	Usually reduced	More often only mildly reduced or preserved[a]
Aetiology	Congestive cardiomyopathy more common	Aortic and mitral valve disease more common[b]
Diagnosis	Easier	More difficult[c]
Treatment provision	Improving	Remains poor[d]
Comorbidities	Less common	More common[e]
Hospitalization	Common	More common[f]
Quality of life	Poor	Worse

Adapted from Reference [8].
[a]See Chapter 2.
[b]See Chapter 4.
[c]See Chapter 5.
[d]See Chapter 6.
[e]See Chapter 8.
[f]See Chapter 12.

differences in the aetiology of heart failure in older and younger patients; they affect disease progression and affect treatment strategies.

- These same changes are partly responsible for the diagnostic difficulties encountered in older patients.

- Evidence that the standard treatments for heart failure are safe and effective in older patients has been slow to appear, and even slower to be translated into practice. This is reflected in a relative lack of specific advice in published guidelines about their management.

- Some relatively young patients have comorbidities, which adversely affect disease progression, treatment and/or the quality of life. However, multiple comorbidities are the norm for older patients.

- Heart failure is now the commonest cause of admission to hospital in the aging population.

- The quality of life is poor for all patients, but more so for those who are older.

- Providing acceptable end of life care for older patients is more complex and time consuming.

Each of these issues is addressed in the following chapters.

1.5   The level of evidence for treating older patients

Many of the recommendations – and much of the advice – for the treatment and management of heart failure which is provided in published guidelines is based on meta-analyses of randomized controlled trials. The level of evidence for much of this advice is graded as 1++ to 1− [4]: older patients were excluded from most of these studies (see Chapter 6). Consequently, much of the advice given in this book cannot be based directly on the landmark randomized controlled trials as it is for younger patients. It is therefore based on:

- Subgroup analyses from these reports

- Other studies from which older patients were not excluded

- Studies specifically of older patients

- Examples of recommended best practice based on the clinical experience of experts in the field.

International and national guidelines classify this level of evidence (Table 1.2) mostly as level 2+ to 4, and recommendations based on such evidence is graded as C and D [4]. Basing advice on this level of evidence is clearly less compelling than that of levels 1++ to 1−, but it should be noted that up to 40% of the evidence presented in published guidelines is similarly graded [4].

Table 1.2   Grading of levels of evidence and of recommendations [4].

Levels of evidence
    2+ Well-conducted case control or cohort studies with a low risk of confounding or bias and a moderate probability that the relationship is causal.
    2 Case control or cohort studies with a high risk of confounding or bias and a significant risk that the relationship is not causal.
    3 Nonanalytic studies, for example case reports, case series.
    4 Expert opinion.
Grade of recommendations
    C A body of evidence including studies rated as 2+ , directly applicable to the target population and demonstrating overall consistency of results; *or*
    Extrapolated evidence from studies rated as 2++

    D Evidence level 3 or 4; *or*
    Extrapolated evidence from studies rated as 2+

References

1. Poole-Wilson, P.A. (1997) History, definition and classification of heart failure, in *Heart Failure* (eds P.A. Poole-Wilson, W.S. Colucci, B.M. Massie *et al.*), Churchill Livingstone, Ch. 19, pp. 269–295.
2. American College of Cardiology/American Heart Association (2005) Guideline update for the diagnosis and management of chronic heart failure in the adult. *Circulation*, **112**, 154–235.
3. Swedberg, K., Cleland, J., Dargie, H. *et al.* (2005) Guidelines for the diagnosis and treatment of chronic heart failure: full text (update 2005). The Task Force for the diagnosis and treatment of CHF of the European Society of Cardiology. *European Heart Journal*, **26**, 1115–1140.
4. Scottish Intercollegiate Guidelines Network (SIGN) (1995) Management of chronic heart failure. A national clinical guideline. Royal College of Physicians, Edinburgh. Available at www.sign.ac.uk.
5. *Concise Oxford English Dictionary* (2005), Oxford University Press.
6. Craft, N. (2005) *The Contribution of Increasing Life Expectancy to the Growth of Living Standards in the UK 1870–2001*, School of Economics, London.
7. Batchelor, W.B., Jollis, J.G. and Friesinger, G.C. (1999) The challenge of health care delivery to elderly patients with cardiovascular disease. *Cardiology Clinics*, **17**, 1–15.
8. Rich, M.W. (2005) Office management of heart failure in the elderly. *American Journal of Medicine*, **118**, 342–348.

2
Epidemiology

Christopher Ward

Ninewells Hospital and Medical School, Dundee

Key messages

- Epidemiological studies highlight important clinical, administrative and financial implications of heart failure in older people.

- The prevalence of heart failure increases with age: 80% of patients are aged 65 years or older.

- The age-related increase in prevalence is predominantly an increase in the number of female patients.

- One half of older patients with heart failure have preserved left ventricular systolic function.

- The prognosis of heart failure worsens with increasing age.

- As life expectancy increases so will the prevalence of heart failure.

2.1   Epidemiology, demography and prognosis

The reported prevalence of heart failure is affected by numerous factors, especially local demographics, the patients' age and gender, whether the study was based on hospitalized or community patients, and on the diagnostic criteria used. Notably, with respect to the latter point, prevalence is affected by whether or not patients

A Practical Guide to Heart Failure in Older People, Edited by C Ward and M D Witham
© 2009 John Wiley & Sons, Ltd

with preserved left ventricular systolic function (HF-PSF) were included in addition to those with left ventricular systolic dysfunction (HF-LVSD) (see below). Despite these confounding factors it is now generally agreed that the overall prevalence of heart failure in westernized countries is in the region of 20 per 1000 population [1].

2.2   Heart failure with preserved left ventricular systolic function (HF-PSF) (see also Chapter 5)

The concept of HF-PSF is important both epidemiologically and clinically. Until 30 years ago [2], it was assumed that heart failure was always caused by left ventricular systolic dysfunction, but today – following a protracted debate – it is agreed that several pathological processes, including myocardial hypertrophy, fibrosis or infiltration, can reduce the ability of the ventricle to fill normally during diastole because the myocardium becomes 'stiff'. This process reaches a point where the heart is unable to provide the necessary cardiac output to support normal body functions [3, 4]. In these situations therefore, heart failure does not occur because the left ventricle is 'weak' in the usual sense of the term.

Epidemiologically, and in some respects clinically, HF-PSF is distinct from HF-LVSD [4].

Epidemiological studies of heart failure prior to the acceptance of HF-PSF have, in retrospect, given an inaccurate picture of heart failure. They fall into three groups:

1.   In studies reported prior to its being recognized, and when the diagnosis of heart failure was based primarily on clinical criteria, some patients with HF-PSF and with HF-LVSD were included (as were some with neither), whereas others were not.

2.   During the same period, but following the introduction of echocardiography, patients with HF-PSF were excluded because, by definition, they did not have a reduced left ventricular ejection fraction which was at that time a prerequisite for diagnosing heart failure.

3.   The same is true of epidemiological data based on information from major drug trials. Echocardiographic evidence of reduced left ventricular systolic function was usually a criterion for inclusion.

It is only recently that epidemiologists have been able to provide an overview of heart failure and to identify differences between the two patterns of left ventricular dysfunction.

Now, despite some overlap between the reported characteristics of the two groups (HF-LVSD and HF-PSF) because of nonuniformity of case selection and diagnostic criteria, several important differences have been identified [4–7]:

- Patients with HF-PSF make up 40–50% of the heart failure population [1] and are 1–5 years older than those with LVSD.

- The majority (51–84%) are female.

- There is a high prevalence of hypertension in patients with HF-PSF (57–84%) and as a result, left ventricular hypertrophy is common.

- Up to 30% of cases of post-myocardial infarction heart failure have HF-PSF, probably resulting from recurrent silent myocardial ischaemia leading to patchy fibrosis [8] (see Chapter 4).

- Aortic stenosis is present in 10–33% of patients with HF-PSF, but in only 5–12% with HF-LVSD [9, 10].

- Comorbidities, including atrial fibrillation, are more common than in HF-LVSD.

Yet, debate persists regarding the prognosis of HF-PSF compared to that of LVSD [4] and often, as with other aspects of epidemiology, it is because of a nonuniformity of study design. However, most reports describe a better prognosis for those with HF-PSF, sometimes recording that the annual mortality is only half that of patients with LVSD [3, 11, 12].

The overall findings of these epidemiological studies have three important consequences. First, the age-related increase in the prevalence of heart failure is predominantly an increase in those with HF-PSF. Second, as life expectancy increases, so the percentage of cases with HF-PSF will increase further. Third, because the majority of patients with HF-PSF are female, the increasing burden of heart failure will affect predominantly the female population (see Figures 2.1a and b).

2.3 Prevalence, incidence and prognosis

The 'ball park' figure, that 20/1000 adults have heart failure [1], obscures the dramatic impact that age has on its prevalence.

The prevalence increases almost exponentially from approximately 2/1000 in people aged less than 55 years to 10/1000 in those aged 50–59 years [14], and to 90–100/1000 in those aged 80–90 years [15–18]. In some reports, the increasing prevalence is described in different terms: as increasing by 27% per decade increase

(a)

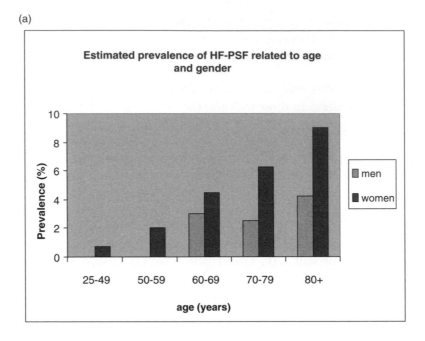

(b)

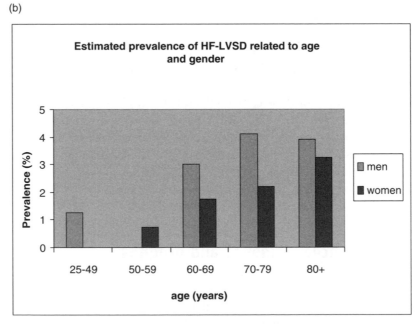

Figure 2.1 Relationship between age and gender. (a) For HF-PSF patients; (b) For HF-LVSD patients. HF-PSF is more common in women in all age groups and HF-LVSD in men in all age groups. (Based on Ref. [13].)

in age in men and by 61% in women [19], and as doubling each decade after the age of 45 [18,20].

Between 78 and 87% of patients are aged over 65 years [16, 20] of whom 60% are older than 75 years: this age (75 years) is reported as the average age at the time of diagnosis [16, 19, 21].

Similarly, in the USA, 80% of patients are aged 65 years or older [22].

There is a comparable age-related increase in incidence: from 2.0–2.5/1000 per year below the age of 60 to approximately 30–40/1000 year in the over-80s. As with prevalence, this represents a doubling of the number of cases each decade [14, 18, 23, 24].

The reported prevalence and incidence of heart failure in men compared to that in women depends to a significant extent on whether or not cases with HF-PSF were included, and on the age of patients studied. HF-PSF becomes increasingly common in women as they age, due largely to their higher prevalence of hypertension. This is reflected in some (but not all) reports describing the prevalence of heart failure in women as increasingly exceeding that in men after the age of 60 years [13, 24, 25].

The age-related increase in prevalence and incidence has been reported from the UK, the USA and from continental Europe (see Figures 2.2–2.6).

The age-related increase in prevalence and incidence is explained by the lifelong progressive natural history of cardiovascular disease and of hypertension, and by their interaction with the cardiovascular changes attributed to normal aging (see Chapter 3).

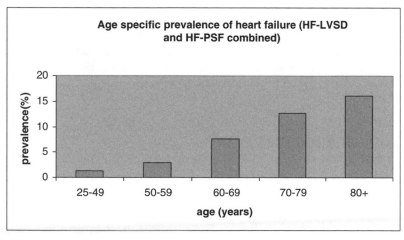

Figure 2.2   The prevalence of heart failure in Europe related to age. (Adapted from Ref. [13].)

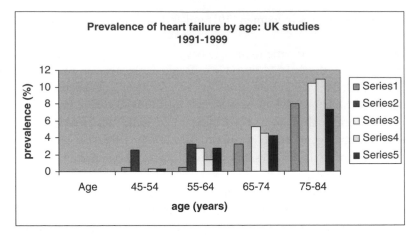

Figure 2.3　The prevalence of heart failure in UK related to age. (Series numbers refer to different UK studies detailed in Ref. [26]). Despite considerable variation in the reported prevalence, each study shows that prevalence increases with age.

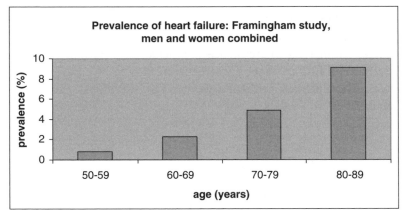

Figure 2.4　The prevalence (%) of heart failure in USA related to age. Adapted from Ref. [14]. (The low prevalence reported in this study, which was approximately half that reported in Ref. [13], can be at least partly attributed to the fact that diagnostic criteria in this study did not include echocardiography.)

2.4　Age and prognosis

The treatment now available for heart failure has improved life expectancy in all age groups (see Chapter 6) but, with very few exceptions, optimum treatment – even in low-risk patients – is palliative rather than curative. The ability to assess prognosis is important in order to test the efficacy of new treatments, to target those patients in whom it is worse than average, and to inform the patients and their carers.

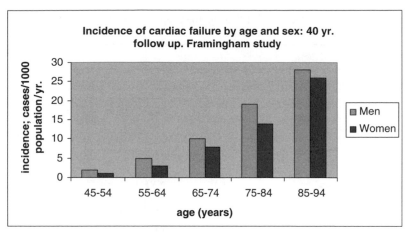

Figure 2.5 Incidence of cardiac failure by age and gender: 40-year follow-up. (Adapted from Ref. [18].)

Many attempts have been made to identify specific tests that reliably predict the prognosis and which identify these high-risk patients, but none does so consistently [26]. This is not surprising. First, the prognosis is dependent on numerous interacting factors, the impact of which varies between patients. Second, one of the objectives of seeking predictive tests has been to use them to assess the life expectancy of individual patients. This has led to the development of prognostic models in which a numerical score is given to each of a number of variable risk factors. As might be expected, the most accurate predictive models are the most impractical to use because of the numerous variables which must be taken into account to calculate the score [27, 28].

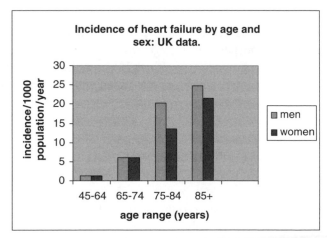

Figure 2.6 Incidence of heart failure by age and gender: UK data. (Based on Ref. [24].) (Data from general practices in Scotland 1999–2000.)

Table 2.1 Selected variables which affect the prognosis (positively or negatively) in heart failure.

Variable	
Patient characteristic/comorbidities	Age
	Gender
	Heart failure aetiology
	Diabetes[a]
	Renal dysfunction[a]
	Anaemia[a]
	Depression[a]
Functional status	NYHA class
Ventricular size/function	6 min walk test
	Ejection fraction
	LV dimensions
Results of investigations	BNP
	Cholesterol
	ECG bundle branch block
	Chest X-ray cardiothoracic ratio
Prescribed medicines	ACE inhibitor
	Beta blocker
	Aldosterone receptor blocker
	Statin

Adapted from Ref. [27].
[a]Factors more common in older patients.

The most easily assessed factors which have a bearing on the prognosis can usefully be classified under four broad headings [27] (Table 2.1). Most of the patient characteristics which are included are more common in older patients and, in conjunction with the effects on the cardiovascular system of 'normal' aging (see Chapter 3), largely explain the high mortality in this age group.

Most of the listed factors – and many others [26] – reflect, to a greater or lesser extent, one of four key markers which are associated with a worsening prognosis:

- Advanced age
- Left ventricular size and function
- Symptom severity and chronicity
- The impact of comorbidities

Studies which do not take equal account of these factors provide very different estimates of the prognosis in heart failure [29]. Nevertheless, 'ball park' figures which are still commonly quoted are that approximately 50% of patients with New York Heart Association (NYHA) class IV symptoms (see Table 2.2), despite optimal medication, die within a year, and that 50% of the remainder die within 5 years [30, 31].

Table 2.2 New York Heart Association functional classification of heart failure.

Class	Patient status
I	No limitation of normal physical activity
II	Comfortable at rest but limited in normal daily activity
III	Comfortable at rest but marked limitation of physical activity
IV	Symptomatic at rest or with minimal activity

More recent studies quote the mortality as 30–40% within a year of diagnosis and 65% after 5 years [15, 16]. Not surprisingly, the mortality rate is higher in older than in younger patients; however, with increasing age the rise in mortality appears in some reports to be greater than the rise in prevalence, being variously described as increasing by 10–25% per decade or as doubling during the same time period (Table 2.3; see also Figure 2.2). This does not necessarily mean that advancing age *per se* is responsible for the worsening prognosis, as the prevalence of comorbidities also increase with age (Table 2.4; see also Chapter 8).

Table 2.3 The effect of age on mortality.

Author [Reference]	Calculated increase in risk
McIntyre *et al.* [21]	In patients aged <55, 1 year mortality 24.2% aged >84 58.1%
Martinez-Selles *et al.* [32]	In patients aged <75, 1 year mortality 23.5% aged >75 34.1%
Pulignano *et al.* [33]	Mortality increase 2.8% per year
Pocock *et al.* [34]	HR 1.73/decade over age 60
Senni *et al.* [35]	RR 1.047 per year increase in age

HR = Hazard Ratio. RR = Relative Risk.

Table 2.4 Selected prognostic variables with a calculated Hazard Ratio >1.25. (Based on Ref. [34] with modification.)

Age
Insulin-dependent diabetes
Non-insulin-dependent diabetes
NYHA class III/IV
Renal dysfunction
Current smoking
ECG: bundle branch block
Hospitalization within 6/12 months
Prior myocardial infarction
Symptom duration >2 years

2.5   The effects of gender and race on prevalence and prognosis

Gender

As with other aspects of the epidemiology of heart failure, the reported impact of gender on prevalence and prognosis is influenced by the demographic variables of the patient cohort studied, and on the diagnostic criteria. In broad terms, the prevalence in male and female patients is similar, but this disguises the fact that there are significant age-related gender differences. The prevalence of heart failure appears to be higher in men before the age of 70 years and in women thereafter (see Figures 2.1a and b).

The higher prevalence in older women is attributed to three main factors: (i) they have a greater life expectancy (see below); (ii) the prevalence of hypertension is higher in older women (as noted above); and (iii) women are more likely to develop left ventricular hypertrophy (and therefore to develop heart failure) in response to hypertension, diabetes and obesity than are men – perhaps because of a reduction in the protective effect of oestrogens following the menopause [36].

Yet, although heart failure is more common in women, their survival is significantly better than that of men, and this is independent of age and irrespective of disease severity [37].

Race

The epidemiology of heart failure in African Americans in the USA and in subjects from the Indian subcontinent in the UK is different from that of their respective white compatriots.

In 2005, African Americans (12.8%) and Hispanics (14.4%) comprised approximately 25% of the USA population, but it is predicted that by 2050 Hispanics will account for 30% [38]. Major differences between the racial groups therefore have important implications for clinicians and for service planning:

- The prevalence of heart failure is higher in African Americans than in the white and Hispanic populations (approximately 3% versus 2%) [39].

- African Americans develop symptoms at a younger age and the mortality is higher – by a factor of 1.8 in male subjects and by 2.4 in female subjects [40].

- Unlike in their white counterparts, hypertension is the principal cause of heart failure in African Americans, and appears to run a particularly aggressive course [39, 41–43].

- Epidemiological data regarding the prevalence of heart failure in the Hispanic population are conflicting [44, 45]. However, because of the high prevalence of cardiovascular risk factors in this group (notably diabetes), it seems inevitable that the prevalence of heart failure will be comparably high.

The largest ethnic groups of UK citizens are from the Indian subcontinent (Southern Asia) and comprise 4% of the population, almost half of whom live in London and the South East. African and Caribbean citizens account for 2% of the UK population.
There are important epidemiological differences between South Asian, African Caribbean and the indigenous UK populations:

- The prevalence of coronary artery disease in South Asians is approximately 40% higher than in the indigenous population [46], but the risk of developing heart failure in the 60–79 age group is fivefold higher [47]; the symptoms also develop several years sooner [48].

- These dramatic differences are probably due to a combination of a fourfold higher prevalence of type 2 diabetes and of the metabolic syndrome and, to a lesser extent, an increase in the prevalence of conventional risk factors. Afro-Caribbeans in the UK have a threefold higher risk of developing heart failure than the indigenous population, but have a lower prevalence of coronary artery disease.

- As in African Americans, the high prevalence of heart failure is explained by the comparably high prevalence of hypertension.

2.6 The increasing prevalence of heart failure and longevity

Heart failure is not only common, it is increasingly so [49], and there are two main reasons for this. The first reason, paradoxically, is related to improvements in the treatment of the commonest causes of heart failure, coronary artery disease and hypertension. Thrombolysis has reduced the mortality from myocardial infarction, but does not necessarily salvage all of the infarcted myocardium, and medication has reduced the incidence of strokes caused by hypertension. However, in each situation the underlying hypertension or coronary artery-related vascular disease persists. Consequently, many survivors subsequently succumb to the long-term effects of these pathologies on myocardial function [49].
The second reason is that life expectancy is improving [50]:

- In the UK, life expectancy at birth has increased from approximately 71 years in men and 77 years in women in 1981, to 76 and 80 years respectively in 2001 [50].

- Men aged 65 in 2005 can expect on average to live to almost 82, almost 4 years longer than those born in 1981; the respective data for women are to live to 84.5 years, some 2.5 years longer [50] (Figure 2.7).

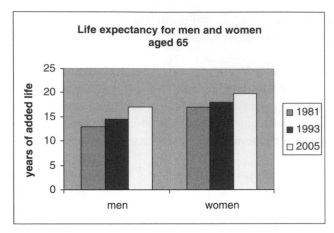

Figure 2.7   The improving life expectancy for men and women aged 65, between 1981 and 2005. (Based on data from Ref. [50].)

- It has been estimated that by 2051, men aged 65 can expect to live a further 22 years and women a further 24 years.

- As a result of this trend it is estimated that the percentage of the population aged >85 will double in the next 30 years.

- Similarly, in the USA the percentage of the population aged over 80 years is predicted to treble in the next 50 years [51].

And, as life expectancy improves so too will the prevalence of heart failure increase because it is age-related.

2.7   The implications of epidemiological and demographic data

The current and predicted epidemiological and demographic data have serious implications for health care provision and funding. While healthy life expectancy (years spent in good or fairly good health) has increased, so has the time spent in poor health – partly because of improved treatments for acute cardiovascular events and heart failure. In the twenty years to 2001, the time spent in poor health increased from 10.1 to 11.6 years in women and from 6.5 to 8.7 years in men. Heart failure is an increasingly prevalent contributing factor to the years spent in poor health.

It has been estimated that the number of cases of heart failure will almost double between 1996 and 2026 in the 65–75-year age group, and during the same period will almost treble in the over-75s [52]. This will place additional burden on health care facilities, which in many countries are inadequate to deal optimally even with current patient numbers.

Estimates of the cost of caring for patients vary widely [53], but a number of relevant observations are well documented:

- In westernized countries, 1–2% of health care expenditure is for the care of patients with heart failure [54].

- A characteristic of older patients with heart failure is that they are often hospitalized (see Chapter 12).

- In many countries the cost of caring for hospitalized patients accounts for 65–75% of all health care expenditure [55].

- A significant proportion of the cost of caring for older patients is for the management of the comorbidities which often accompany heart failure (see Chapter 8).

- The annual cost of caring for patients aged 75–84 is more than two- to threefold that for those aged between 54 and 74 years: of these costs, 60% is spent on inpatient care [56].

- The old-age dependency ratio, (the number of people above pensionable age as a proportion of the number of people of working age) increased from approximately 20% in the 1960s to approximately 27% between 1980 and 2003, and is projected to rise to 47% by 2051 [50, 52].

- Over the next few decades therefore, these increasing costs are likely to fall on a (relatively) declining work force.

In a UK study, the cost of heart failure care as a percentage of the total health care expenditure [54, 57] was estimated (1995 data) to be £628.6 million [26]. This represented 1.83% of the total health care expenditure, rising over 5 years to 1.91% by 2000, and does not include the very substantial costs of nursing home care [57].

The increasing financial burden of treating heart failure can be partially offset by:

- Using existing strategies for the primary prevention of heart failure in high-risk patients (see Chapters 6 and 9).

- Optimizing treatment (see Chapter 6).

- Reducing hospitalization (see Chapter 12).

References

1. McMurray, J., Komadja, M., Anker, S. and Gardner, R. (2006) Heart failure: epidemiology, pathophysiology and diagnosis, in *The European Society of Cardiology Textbook of Cardiovascular Medicine* (eds J.A. Cramm, T.F. Luscher and P.W. Serryus), Blackwell Publishing, pp. 685–720.
2. Dodek, A., Kassemaum, D.G. and Larson, M.G. (1972) Pulmonary oedema in coronary artery disease without cardiomegaly. Paradox of the stiff heart. *New England Journal of Medicine*, **286**, 1347–1350.
3. Zile, M.R. and Brutsaert, D.L. (2002) New concepts of diastolic dysfunction and diastolic heart failure: Diagnosis, prognosis, and measurement of diastolic function. *Circulation*, **105**, 1387–1393.
4. Owan, T.E. and Redfield, M.M. (2005) Epidemiology of diastolic heart failure. *Progress in Cardiovascular Disease*, **47** (5), 320–332.
5. Varsan, R.S. and Levy, D. (2000) Defining diastolic heart failure: A call for standardised diagnostic criteria. *Circulation*, **101** (17), 2118–2121.
6. Hogg, K., Swedberg, K. and McMurray, J. (2004) Heart failure with preserved left ventricular systolic function: Epidemiology, clinical characteristics and prognosis. *Journal of the American College of Cardiology*, **43**, 317–327.
7. Kitzman, D.W., Little, W.C., Brubaker, P.H. *et al.* (2002) Pathophysiological characterisation of isolated diastolic heart failure in comparison to systolic heart failure. *Journal of the American Medical Association*, **288**, 2144–2150.
8. Hellermann, J.P., Jacobsen, S.J., Reeder, G.S. *et al.* (2003) Heart failure after myocardial infarction: Prevalence of preserved left ventricular systolic function in the community. *American Heart Journal*, **145**, 742–748.
9. Berry, C., Hogg, K., Norrie, J. *et al.* (2005) Heart failure with preserved left ventricular function: a hospital cohort study. *Heart*, **91**, 907–913.
10. Valera-Roman, A., Grigorian, I., Barge, E. *et al.* (2005) Heart failure with preserved and deteriorated left ventricular ejection fraction. *Heart*, **91**, 489–494.
11. Franklin, K.M. and Aurigemma, G.P. (2005) Prognosis in diastolic heart failure. *Progress in Cardiovascular Diseases*, **47**, 333–339.
12. Haney, S., Sur, D. and Xu, Z. (2005) Diastolic heart failure: A review and primary care perspective. *Journal of the American Board of Family Practice*, **18**, 189–198.
13. Ciea, F., Fonsecca, C., Mota, T. *et al.* (2002) Prevalence of chronic heart failure in Southwestern Europe: The EPICA study. *European Journal of Heart Failure*, **4**, 531–539.
14. Kannel, W.B. and Belanger, A.J. (1991) Epidemiology of heart failure. *American Heart Journal*, **121**, 951–957.
15. Bleumink, G.S., Knetsch, A.M., McAlister, F.A. *et al.* (2004) Quantifying the heart failure epidemic: prevalence, incidence rate, lifetime risk and prognosis of heart failure. The Rotterdam Study. *European Heart Journal*, **25**, 1614–1619.
16. Cowie, M.R., Wood, D.A., Coates, A.J.S. *et al.* (1999) Incidence and aetiology of heart failure: A population-based study. *European Heart Journal*, **20**, 421–428.

17. McMurray, J.J. and Stewart, S. (2000) Epidemiology, aetiology and prognosis of heart failure. *Heart*, **83**, 596–602.
18. Kannel, W.B. (2000) Incidence and epidemiology of heart failure. *Heart Failure Reviews*, **5**, 167–173.
19. Ho, K.K., Anderson, K.M., Kannel, W.B. *et al.* (1993) Survival after the onset of heart failure in the Framingham Heart Study subjects. *Circulation*, **88**, 107–115.
20. Rich, M.W. (1997) Epidemiology, pathophysiology and etiology of congestive heart failure in older adults. *Journal of the American Geriatric Society*, **45**, 968–974.
21. MacIntyre, K., Capewell, S., Stewart, S. *et al.* (2000) Evidence of improving prognosis of heart failure. *Circulation*, **102**, 1126–1131.
22. Gillum, R.F. (1993) Epidemiology of heart failure in the United States. *American Heart Journal*, **126**, 1042–1047.
23. van Jaarsveld, C.H.M., Ranchor, A.V., Kempen, G.I.J.M. *et al.* (2006) Epidemiology of heart failure in a community-based study of subjects aged =/> 57 years: Incidence and longterm survival. *European Journal of Heart Failure*, **8**, 23–30.
24. Murphy, N.F., Simpson, C.R., McAlister, F.A. *et al.* (2004) National survey of the prevalence, incidence, primary care burden and treatment of heart failure in Scotland. *Heart*, **90**, 1129–1136.
25. Mair, F.S., Crowley, T.S. and Bundred, P.E. (1996) Prevalence, aetiology and management of heart failure in general practice. *British Journal of General Practice*, **46**, 77–79.
26. British Heart Foundation Health Promotion Research Group (2006) *Coronary Heart Disease Statistics* (ed. P. Weissbeg), British Heart Foundation, 14 Fitzhardinge Street, London, W1H 6DH (www.heartstats.org).
27. Mosterd, A. and Hoes, A.W. (2007) Clinical epidemiology of heart failure. *Heart*, **93**, 1137–1146.
28. Levy, W.C., Mozaffarian, D., Linker, S.T. *et al.* (2006) The Seattle heart failure model: prediction of survival in heart failure. *Circulation*, **113**, 1424–1433.
29. Clelland, J.G.F. and Clarke, A. (1999) Has the survival of the heart failure population changed? Lessons from trials. *American Journal of Cardiology*, **83**, 112D–119D.
30. McMurray, J., McDonagh, T., Morrison, T.C. and Dargie, H.J. (1993) Trends in hospitalisation for heart failure in Scotland 1980–1990. *European Heart Journal*, **14**, 1158–1162.
31. Clelland, J.G.F., Gemmell, I., Khand, A. and Boddy, A. (1999) Is the prognosis of heart failure improving? *European Journal of Heart Failure*, **1**, 229–241.
32. Martinez-Selles, M., Robles, J.A.G., Prieto, L. *et al.* (2005) Heart failure in the elderly: age-related differences in clinical profile and mortality. *International Journal of Cardiology*, **102**, 55–60.
33. Pulignano, G., Del Sindaco, D., Tavazzi, L. *et al.* (2002) Clinical features and outcomes of elderly outpatients with heart failure followed up in hospital cardiology units: Data from a large nationwide cardiology database (IN-CHF Register). *American Heart Journal*, **143**, 45–55.
34. Pocock, S.J., Wang, D., Pfeffer, M.A. *et al.* (2006) Predictors of mortality and morbidity in patients with chronic heart failure. *European Heart Journal*, **27**, 65–75.

35. Senni, M., Tribouilloy, C.M., Rodeheffer, R.J. *et al.* (1999) Congestive heart failure in the community: Trends in incidence and survival in a 10-year period. *Archives of Internal Medicine*, **159**, 29–34.

36. Regitz-Zagrosec, V., Brokat, B. and Tschope, C. (2007) Role of gender in heart failure with normal left ventricular ejection fraction. *Progress in Cardiovascular Diseases*, **49**, 241–251.

37. Adams, K.F., Sueta, C.A., Gheorghiade, M. *et al.* (1999) Gender differences in survival in advanced heat failure: Insights from the FIRST study. *Circulation*, **99**, 1816–1821.

38. US Census Bureau: http://www.census.gov/statab/www/poprace.html (accessed December 2004).

39. Yancy, W.C. (2000) Heart failure in African Americans: A cardiovascular enigma. *Journal of Cardiac Failure*, **6**, 183–193.

40. Exner, D.V., Dreis, D.L., Domanski, M.J. *et al.* (2001) Lesser response to angiotensin converting inhibitor enzyme inhibitor therapy in black as compared with white patients with left ventricular dysfunction. *New England Journal of Medicine*, **344**, 1351–1357.

41. Yancy, C.W. (2005) Heart failure in African Americans. *American Journal of Cardiology*, (96 suppl), 3i–12i.

42. Philbin, E.F., Weil, H.F.C., Francis, C.A. *et al.* (2000) Race-related differences among patients with left ventricular dysfunction: Observations from a biracial angiographic cohort. *Journal of Cardiac Failure*, **6**, 187–193.

43. Ferdinand, K.C. (2007) African American heart failure trial: Role of endothelial dysfunction and heart failure in African Americans. *American Journal of Cardiology*, (99 suppl), 3D–6D.

44. Swenson, C.J., Trepka, M.J., Rewers, M.J. *et al.* (2002) Cardiovascular disease mortality in Hispanic and Non-Hispanic Whites. *American Journal of Epidemiology*, **156**, 919–928.

45. Hunt, K.J., Resendez, R.G., Williams, K. *et al.* (2003) All-cause cardiovascular mortality among Mexican-Americans and non-Hispanic white older participants in the San Antonio heart study – evidence against the "Hispanic Paradox". *American Journal of Epidemiology*, **158**, 1048–1057.

46. Bhopal, R. (2000) What is the risk of coronary artery disease in south Asians? A review of UK research. *Journal of Public Health Medicine*, **22**, 375–385.

47. Chaturvedi, N. (2003) Ethnic differences in cardiovascular disease. *Heart*, **89**, 681–686.

48. Blackledge, H.M., Newton, J. and Squires, I.B. (2003) Prognosis for south Asians and white patients newly admitted to hospital with heart failure in the United Kingdom: historical cohort study. *British Medical Journal*, **327**, 526–530.

49. Ghali, J.K., Cooper, R. and Ford, E. (1990) Trends in hospitalisation rates for heart failure in the United States, 1973–1986. Evidence for increasing population prevalence. *Archives of Internal Medicine*, **150**, 769–773.

50. Office of National Statistics: www.statistics.gov.uk.

51. Batchelor, W.B., Jollis, J.G. and Friesinger, G.C. (1999) The challenge of health care delivery to elderly patients with cardiovascular disease. *Cardiology Clinics*, **17** (1), 1–15.

52. Kelly, D.T. (1997) Our future society: A global challenge. *Circulation*, **95**, 2459–2464.

53. Liao, L., Anstrom, K.J., Gottdiener, J.S. *et al.* (2007) Long-term costs and resource use in elderly participants, with congestive heart failure in the Cardiovascular Health Study. *American Heart Journal*, **153**, 245–252.

54. Harlan, W.R. (1989) Economic considerations that influence health policy and research. *Hypertension*, **13** (Suppl 1), 1:158–1:163.

55. McMurray, J., Hart, W. and Rhodes, G. (1993) An evaluation of the cost of heart failure to the National Health Service in the UK. *British Journal of Medical Economics*, **6**, 99–110.

56. Stewart, S., Jenkins, A., Buchan, S. *et al.* (2002) The current cost of heart failure to the National Health Service in the UK. *European Journal of Heart Failure*, **4**, 361–371.

57. Stewart, S. (2005) Financial aspects of heart failure programmes of care. *European Journal of Heart Failure*, **7**, 423–428.

3

Heart failure and the aging heart

Helen Oxenham

Cardiology Department Borders General Hospital, Melrose, Roxburghshire

---

Key Messages

- Clinical and subclinical cardiovascular disease are more common in older than in younger people.

- Normal cardiovascular aging causes systolic hypertension and impaired left ventricular diastolic function. As a result, the aging heart is unable to respond normally to physiological demands and to myocardial damage.

- These phenomena largely explain the natural history and prevalence of heart failure in older people.

3.1   Introduction

The epidemiology and aetiology of heart failure in older patients are discussed in Chapters 2 and 4, respectively. They describe important differences between older and younger patients:

- The prevalence of heart failure increases incrementally from the sixth decade of life onwards [1, 2].

- The majority of older patients with heart failure have preserved left ventricular systolic function [3].

A Practical Guide to Heart Failure in Older People, Edited by C Ward and M D Witham
© 2009 John Wiley & Sons, Ltd

- Atrial fibrillation is more common in older patients, in whom it is more likely to precipitate acute heart failure.

- Older patients are more likely to develop heart failure following myocardial infarction.

- The prognosis of heart failure is worse in older patients.

In this chapter we explore the underlying reasons for these observations.

   The development and natural history of heart failure in older patients can be largely explained by the interaction of a number of different pathological and physiological processes:

1. The prevalence of overt and subclinical cardiovascular disease in older people.

2. Age-related changes in cardiovascular structure and function.

3. Noncardiovascular age-related changes.

4. The effect of age on the cardiovascular responses to exercise and to physiological stress.

5. The pathogenesis of heart failure.

6. The responses of the aging cardiovascular system to heart failure.

3.2   Overt and subclinical cardiovascular disease in older people

The dramatic increase in the prevalence of coronary artery disease, hypertension and valvular disease between the ages of 50 and 80 can be largely explained by the lifelong progression of subclinical atherosclerosis and the subsequent development of clinically overt disease.

Atheroma

The earliest pathological changes of arterial disease – intimal fatty streaks – are present in adolescence and progress throughout life.

   Aging is subsequently associated with:

- an increased thickness of the arterial intima

- hypertrophy of the vascular smooth muscle

- fragmentation of the internal elastic membrane

- an increase in the amount of collagen and collagen crosslinking in the arterial walls [4, 5]

- progressive dilatation and elongation of the major arteries

- increased arterial thickening and stiffness [5].

These changes, and the development of cholesterol-rich atheromatous plaques, progress due to a lifetime exposure to endothelial damage caused by smoking, free radicals, hypercholesterolaemia, diabetes and hypertension. As a result, the severity and extent of clinical and subclinical atheroma increase with age [6–8]. This goes a long way towards explaining the age-related increase in the prevalence of the clinical consequences of plaque development, notably myocardial infarction, which is, in turn the major determinant of the burden of heart failure on the aging population (Figure 3.1).

Subclinical cardiovascular disease

It is only during the past decade that the prevalence and progression of subclinical cardiovascular disease in older people has been comprehensively investigated. It is now clear that the majority of older people, including those with no history or symptoms of coronary, vascular or hypertensive disease, have evidence of subclinical disease.

In the Cardiovascular Health Study [9] an original cohort of 5201 subjects aged 65 years and above was studied. The patients were evaluated on the basis of a detailed clinical history and examination and noninvasive assessment of the heart and vasculature, including electrocardiography, echocardiography, magnetic resonance imaging (MRI) of the brain, carotid duplex scan, retinal photography and

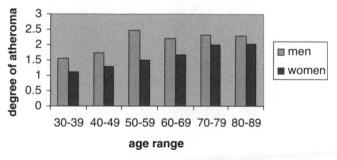

Figure 3.1 Relationship between age and degree of atheroma found at autopsy in men and women. Grade 1 minimal atheroma; grade 3 total vessel occlusion. (Based on data from Refs [7, 8].)

ultrasound of the abdominal aorta [10]. All investigations were repeated at some stage during the study.

Based on 11 years of follow-up:

- Approximately two-thirds of white women and more than three-quarters of white men had either clinical or subclinical cardiovascular disease.

- Half of the women and two-thirds of the men who did not have clinical disease had subclinical disease.

- In men and women without a history of coronary artery disease or hypertension, the prevalence of major ECG changes approximately doubled between the ages of 65 and 85 or older, from 16 to 45.9% and from 10.5 to 31.6%, respectively.

- The prevalence of subclinical noncardiac vascular disease also increased with age: for example, carotid artery stenosis of greater than 50% was present in 4.3% of those aged 65–69, and in 14.3% of those aged over 85. The prevalence of myocardial infarction was fourfold higher in those with severe carotid artery thickening compared to those with minimal thickening.

- Over the 11 years of the study, the incidence of fatal plus nonfatal coronary artery disease in men was 8.2% compared to 4.3% in those with no subclinical disease: the comparable figures in women were 3.8% and 1.5%.

A comparison of heart failure prevalence in older and younger people is provided in Figure 3.2.

The prevalence of clinical and subclinical cardiovascular disease in men and women aged 65 years and older

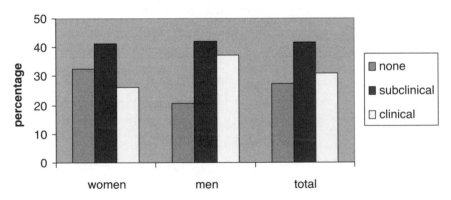

Figure 3.2 The prevalence of clinical and subclinical cardiovascular disease in men and women aged 65 years and older. (Adapted from Ref. [19].)

Aortic and mitral valve disease

The prevalence of aortic and mitral valve disease, the primary aetiology of heart failure in approximately 15% of cases [11], is age-related (see Chapter 4).

More important here is the relationship between these valve pathologies and cardiovascular disease.

Aortic valve disease

The prevalence of the precursors of aortic stenosis, valvular thickening and calcification, increase throughout adult life [12,13].

These progressive aortic valve changes are associated with an increased prevalence of conventional cardiovascular risk factors, and also with an increase in morbidity and mortality from myocardial infarction, angina and stroke [14], the prevalence of each, as noted above, increases almost exponentially with age.

Mitral annular calcification (MAC)

MAC shares several features in common with the aortic sclerosis and stenosis of older patients:

- The prevalence and severity increases with age.

- The conventional risk factors that govern the development and progression of coronary artery and cerebrovascular disease throughout life also dictate the prevalence and severity of MAC [15].

Thus, the risk factors which are responsible for the increasing prevalence of coronary artery disease in older subjects are also responsible for the high prevalence of valvular disease and of heart failure resulting from it [16, 17].

Overt coronary artery disease

The role of coronary artery disease in the aetiology of heart failure is discussed in detail in Chapter 4:

- The most common cause of heart failure is ischaemic heart disease, usually myocardial infarction [7].

- The prevalence of myocardial infarction increases dramatically between the ages of 45 and 75 [18, 19].

- There are comparable increases in the prevalence of angina and strokes.

- Data from North America suggest that more than 80% of myocardial infarctions occur in the over 65s [20].

- Clinically overt coronary artery disease (documented myocardial infarction, a typical history of angina, sudden cardiac death or angiographic evidence of coronary artery disease) has been identified in 40% of men and women aged over 80 years.

Hypertension

Increasing arterial stiffness, due mainly to intimal thickening, is a feature of aging in western societies, even in the absence of demonstrable cardiovascular disease [21, 22], and is associated with arterial dilatation. This causes an increase in systolic blood pressure [22] and a widening of the pulse pressure (because there is no comparable increase in the diastolic blood pressure). This in turn causes an increase in afterload, the systolic pressure against which the ventricle has to contract. These factors may contribute to the development of the left ventricular hypertrophy commonly found in older patients with hypertension.

- The age-related increase in the prevalence of hypertension is dramatic (see Figure 3.3), and occurs in up to 60% or more of the untreated over 80s [20].

- Hypertension causes or contributes to approximately 50% of cases of heart failure.

- Hypertension is more often the primary cause of heart failure in women than in men [23].

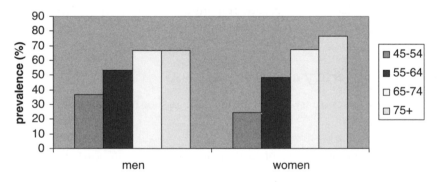

Prevalence of hypertension in middle aged and older people

Figure 3.3 Prevalence of hypertension in middle-aged and older people. Subjects are classified as having high blood pressure if the systolic blood pressure is >140 mmHg, diastolic blood pressure >90 mmHg, or are taking hypotensive medication. (Based on data from Ref. [5].)

3.3   Age-related changes to cardiac structure and function

Significant changes affect the myocardium, arteries and the autonomic nervous system of older healthy volunteers; the same anatomical changes are found in post-mortem examinations of other subjects, and in experimental animals, none of which had demonstrable cardiovascular disease [24, 25]. These studies suggest that age itself, independent of cardiovascular disease, may alter the structure and function of the cardiovascular system (Table 3.1).

Left ventricular (LV) mass

There is an increase in the relative thickness of the LV wall (the ratio of the wall thickness to the chamber radius), but little or no increase in overall LV mass [21]. This latter finding, which seems paradoxical in the light of the increased wall thickness, may be the result of an observed 35% decrease in the total number of myocytes which occurs between the ages of 30 and 70 years. This may in turn be the result of ischaemic injury secondary to a reduction in the number of myocardial capillaries, which has also been noted to occur with increasing age [26, 27]. This dramatic cell loss may be accompanied by a compensatory hypertrophy of the remaining myocytes and an increase in myocardial collagen content [27, 28].

The concentric change in LV shape parallels the age-related arterial stiffening noted above. However, this is different from the changes that occur in hypertension, which often cause not only an increased LV wall thickness but also an associated increase in the LV mass [26]. In other words, these appear to be two distinct processes, and it is likely that the increase in LV mass that is often attributed to the normal aging process is more likely to be predominantly a result of extramyocardial influences such as hypertension, and not to aging *per se*.

There is, surprisingly, no consensus that these changes are accompanied by significant changes in LV volume or systolic function [26, 30].

Left ventricular diastolic function

Diastole is the phase of the cardiac cycle in which there is ventricular relaxation and during which the left ventricle 'stretches' as it fills with blood. Although there are no obvious age-related changes in systolic function, there are dramatic changes in diastolic function which have been identified in more than 85% of healthy people

Table 3.1 Cardiovascular changes attributed to aging, and their consequences.

	Change associated with normal aging	Clinical markers	Clinical consequence(s)
Arterial wall	Increased thickness Reduced compliance	Increased systolic blood pressure, afterload, and pulse wave velocity Widening of pulse pressure Preserved ejection fraction	Hypertension
Myocardium	Loss of myocytes Increased ratio of left ventricular wall thickness to chamber size		
Cellular changes	Reduced sarcoplasmic reticulum, Ca^{2+} ATPase protein concentration Reduced reuptake of Ca^{2+} into sarcoplasmic reticulum	Prolongation of myocardial relaxation Increased isovolumetric relaxation time Reduced left ventricular compliance	Diastolic dysfunction
Systolic function	Preserved ejection fraction Reduced peak strain		Reduced stroke volume on exercise
Diastolic function	Reduced early diastolic filling Increased late diastolic filling Reduced myocardial diastolic velocities	Echocardiographic evidence of: 1. Abnormal LV relaxation; or 2. Abnormal diastolic distension; or 3. Increased diastolic stiffness (see Chapter 5)	Diastolic dysfunction
Renal function	Reduced eGFR		Fluid retention
Pulmonary function	Reduced forced vital capacity (FVC)		Breathlessness

aged over 70 years [31, 32]. These echocardiographically demonstrated structural changes cause increased stiffness of the myocardium which result in:

- A slowing of the normal diastolic relaxation (stretching) of the ventricle.

- A consequent decrease in the rate and volume of ventricular filling.

- This in turn causes a rise in the left ventricular and left atrial pressures [28, 31–34].

These data indicate that, with advancing age, the left ventricle becomes less compliant and has a less effective filling mechanism.

3.4   Other relevant age-related changes

Age-related changes which are relevant to the development of heart failure in older people are not confined to the cardiovascular system; in fact, significant changes also occur in noncardiovascular organs, notably the kidneys, the lungs and in insulin resistance.

Renal function

Renal function declines progressively with advancing age [35]; typically, the glomerular filtration rate (GFR) falls by 25% between the ages of 40 and 65, and continues to do so thereafter [36]. In a study of middle-aged people, an estimated GFR (eGFR) of less than 60 ml min^{-1} predicted a threefold higher incidence of hospitalization because of heart failure than in those whose eGFR was greater than 90 (Hazard Ratio (HR) 1.94; confidence interval (CI) 1.49–2.53). In addition, when heart failure had developed, a substantially greater decline in renal function occurred in those in whom it was previously impaired [37].

Pulmonary function

The forced vital capacity, a measure of usable lung volume, declines progressively with advancing age and may contribute to the clinical presentation of heart failure. Pulmonary function in older people has been shown to be independently associated with increasing LV mass, hypertension and ischaemic heart disease [38]. Some – but not all – of this association is likely to be due to the effects of smoking on both lung function and cardiovascular function. A reduced lung capacity interacts with cardiovascular disease in further reducing exercise capacity.

Insulin resistance

The prevalence of diabetes mellitus increases with age, and is an independent risk factor for the development of heart failure; in fact, it doubles the risk of heart failure occurring in both men and women [38]. Although the cause of this association is unclear, several factors are known to contribute:

- Insulin resistance facilitates atherogenesis [39].

- Diabetes is associated with accelerated myocardial fibrosis, LV hypertrophy and diastolic dysfunction, even in the absence of overt coronary artery disease.

3.5   Responses of the aging cardiovascular system to exercise, normal daily activities and to other physiological stresses

The way in which the cardiovascular system responds to the demands of exercise has similarities to its responses to myocardial damage, in that both require a series of adaptations with a view to increasing the cardiac output.

Responses to physical activity

Normal responses to physical activity

Physical activity requires an increase in cardiac output to supply extra oxygen and nutrients to working muscles. Activation of the autonomic nervous system (adrenergic stimulation) plays a large part in achieving this, by causing:

- an increase in heart rate

- an increase in the force of contraction of the left ventricle

- an increase in the rate at which the ventricle fills during diastole [40]. This occurs because the increased β adrenergic stimulation during exercise accelerates the process of LV relaxation [41].

Physical activity in older people

With advancing age there is a reduced responsiveness to β adrenergic stimulation [42], and this is thought to explain several age-related changes during exercise:

- A reduction in the maximal heart rate [41, 43].

- Reduced myocardial contractility [28] and cardiac output [42].

- A reduction in the volume of blood ejected per beat (stroke volume) at peak exercise [28, 42].

- The age-related impairment in LV diastolic function (as discussed above) results in inadequate ventricular filling, which further limits the cardiac output [29].

These and the other age-related cardiovascular changes discussed above [42–44] are partly responsible for a progressive decline in the level of cardiovascular fitness by 10% per decade [43], as assessed by the maximum oxygen consumption (VO_{2max}), that begins when the subject is in their mid-20s. This is observed particularly in sedentary populations [28], but is less marked in athletes [43] and in older subjects who take regular exercise.

Impaired response of the aging cardiovascular system to other forms of stress

Changes to intravascular volume

Because of the age-related impairment of diastolic function, the noncompliant left ventricle is unable to accommodate rapid increases in intravascular volume. Consequently, pulmonary oedema occurs more readily when older adults receive intravascular fluid.

Decreases in intravascular volume are also poorly tolerated, and significant reductions in stroke volume and cardiac output may follow diuretic or vasodilator therapy in older people, leading to hypotension and underperfusion of the brain and kidneys.

The response of the aging heart to the onset of atrial fibrillation

The prevalence of atrial fibrillation increases with age, and is now thought to be caused by a stretching of the atria [13]. This is attributable to a chronic increase in left atrial pressure and size [46] resulting from the age-related increase in the prevalence of systolic hypertension and the changes in diastolic function, as discussed above. Because of the LV stiffness that results from these changes, adequate ventricular filling is much more dependent on atrial contraction (which contributes 30% to ventricular filling in many older patients) than in younger people. Consequently, ventricular filling – and therefore cardiac output – are dramatically reduced with the onset of atrial fibrillation.

This, combined with a shortened diastolic filling time which occurs because of the rapid ventricular rate in atrial fibrillation, further impairs LV diastolic filling and leads to a further increase in the left atrial pressure. As a result, older people are prone to develop acute heart failure with the onset of atrial fibrillation.

3.6   The pathogenesis of heart failure (see Figure 3.4)

The pathogenesis in younger patients

Myocardial damage, irrespective of the cause, results in a rapid fall in cardiac output and hence a rise in the volume of blood remaining in the (dilated) ventricle. This

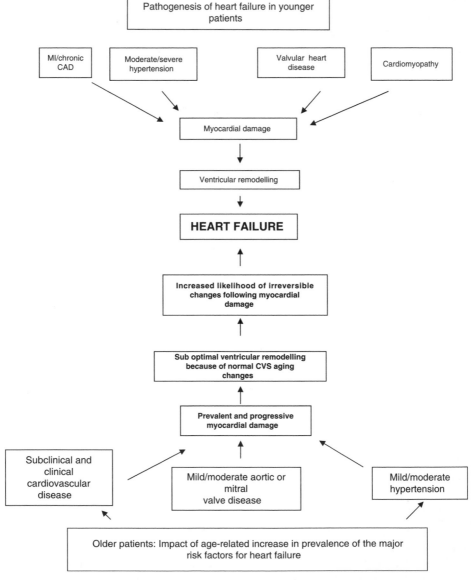

Figure 3.4   The pathogenesis of heart failure in younger and older patients.

promptly triggers the Frank–Starling mechanism ('Starling's law'), which dictates that, up to a point, an increase in myocardial fibre length leads to an increase in the force of contraction.

This is followed by a series of complex inter-related changes to the myocardium, collectively referred to as ventricular remodelling. In essence, these neuroendocrine-driven structural and functional changes are a series of compensatory responses to the damaged muscle and the consequent impaired cardiac function. They are aimed at repairing the damage and restoring and maintaining an adequate circulation. (Detailed reviews of this topic can be found in standard textbooks [47,48].) In summary, the main structural components of the process are:

1.   Expansion ('stretching') of the damaged areas of the myocardium.

2.   Hypertrophy of unaffected myocytes.

3.   Fibrosis of irreparably damaged areas.

The tendency for the cardiac output to fall following myocardial damage triggers the activation of several neurohormonal systems, the best known of which are the renin-angiotensin-aldosterone system (RAAS) and the sympathetic nervous system, both of which help to restore and maintain the cardiac output and blood pressure. This is achieved by a combination of:

•   The maintenance of an adequate GFR (via the RAAS).

•   An increase in the rate and force of contraction of the heart (via the autonomic nervous system).

These and other triggered responses cause an increase in the circulating blood volume into a contracted vascular space, which in turn results in increased venous return to the heart. This leads to further LV dilatation and an augmentation of the force of contraction. However, in the long term these compensatory mechanisms become counterproductive:

•   The more forcefully the heart contracts in response to the Frank–Starling mechanism and beta-adrenergic stimulation, the more it dilates.

•   Continuing LV dilatation is associated with increased ventricular wall stress, and this can only be overcome by a further increase in cardiac work.

•   The continuing activity of the RAAS leads to salt and water retention, and maintains a high peripheral vascular resistance and against which the weakening heart must contract.

Thus, a 'vicious cycle' of progressive heart failure is established.

3.7 The impact of age-related changes to the cardiovascular system on the responses to myocardial damage

The cardiovascular changes that result from aging militate against an optimal response to myocardial damage which, as noted above, include an initial increase in the rate and force of cardiac contraction, hypertrophy of surviving myocytes, and the ability of the left ventricle to promptly dilate and fill during diastole in order to improve cardiac output in response to the Frank–Starling mechanism.

However, because of the age-related loss of myocytes, increasing myocardial stiffness and decrease in beta-adrenergic activity, this does not happen.

These age-related changes help to explain the susceptibility of older patients to develop heart failure, for example following myocardial infarction. They also help to explain the worse prognosis in older patients when heart failure has become established than would be the case with younger patients.

3.8 The prevention of heart failure in older people

As noted in Chapter 2, the prevalence of heart failure is increasing worldwide. Moreover, in the absence of a cure, the reversal of this trend depends on primary and secondary preventions. Evidence summarized above has shown that the majority of older people have clinical or subclinical cardiovascular disease, as a result of which they are at a high risk of developing heart failure.

Older people should therefore be screened for conventional modifiable risk factors and also for evidence of vascular disease (hypertension, angina/myocardial infarction, carotid bruits and claudication). Unfortunately, this topic is not discussed in most standard textbooks, and hence there is limited information available on the benefits of primary preventative strategies in older subjects.

Several points should, however, be noted:

- The SCORE risk assessment programme [49] highlights the importance of addressing all modifiable risk factors.

- There is evidence that an improvement in the lipid profile can significantly reduce cardiovascular risk in older subjects, even within as little as 2–5 years [50].

- The reduction of hypertension, and of LV hypertrophy in older subjects, has a major impact on CVS events.

There is also evidence that a reasonably active lifestyle (see Chapter 7) may effect a reversal or reduction in age-related changes in cardiovascular structure and function:

- Evidence from studies in athletes suggests a slowing or a reduction of some of the age-related changes seen in the cardiovascular system [51].

- Exercise training increases arterial compliance, which may in turn reduce arterial stiffness, independent of any changes in blood pressure [52].

References

1. McDonagh, T.A., Morrison, C.E., Lawrence, A. *et al.* (1997) Symptomatic and asymptomatic left ventricular systolic dysfunction in an urban population. *Lancet*, **350**, 829–833.
2. Kannel, W.B. and Belanger, A.J. (1991) Epidemiology of heart failure. *American Heart Journal*, **121** (3 Pt 1), 951–957.
3. Vasan, R., Larson, M., Benjamin, E. *et al.* (1999) Congestive heart failure in patients with normal versus reduced left ventricular ejection fraction. Prevalence and mortality in a population-based cohort. *Journal of the American College of Cardiology*, **33**, 1948–1955.
4. Joyner, M.J. (2000) Effect of exercise on arterial compliance. *Circulation*, **102**, 1214–1215.
5. Lakatta, E.G. (2000) Cardiovascular aging in health. *Clinics in Geriatric Medicine*, **16**, 419–444.
6. Strong, J.P., Malcom, G.T., McMahan, C.A. *et al.* (1999) Prevalence and extent of atherosclerosis in adolescents and young adults: implications for prevention from the Pathobiological Determinants of Atherosclerosis in Youth Study. *The Journal of the American Medical Association*, **281** (8), 727–735.
7. Ackerman, R.F., Dry, T.J. and Edwards, J.E. (1950) Relationship of various factors to the degree of coronary atherosclerosis in women. *Circulation*, **1**, 1345–1354.
8. White, N.K., Edwards, J.E. and Dry, T.J. (1950) The relationship of the degree of coronary atherosclerosis with age in men. *Circulation*, **1**, 645–654.
9. Kuller, L., Wolf, P., Furberg, C. *et al.* (1994) Prevalence of subclinical atherosclerosis and cardiovascular disease and association with risk factors in the Cardiovascular Health Study. *American Journal of Epidemiology*, **139**, 1164–1179.
10. Kuller, L.H. and Sutton-Tyrrell, K. (1999) Aging and cardiovascular disease. *Cardiology Clinics*, **17** (1), 51–65.
11. Patel, K.R.C., Prince, J., Mirza, S. *et al.* (2008) Evaluation of an open-access heart failure service spanning primary and secondary care. *British Journal of Cardiology*, **15** (1), 35–39.
12. Sahasakul, Y., Edwards, W.D., Naessens, J.M. *et al.* (1988) Age-related changes in aortic and mitral valve thickness: implications for two-dimensional echocardiography based on an autopsy study of 200 normal human hearts. *The American Journal of Cardiology*, **62**, 424–430.
13. Hinchman, D.A. and Otto, C.M. (1999) Valvular disease in the elderly. *Cardiology Clinics*, **17** (1), 137–158.

14. Otto, C.M., Kuusisto, J., Richenbach, D.D. *et al.* (1994) Characterisation of the early lesion of degenerative aortic stenosis – histological and immunohistochemical studies. *Circulation*, **90**, 844–853.

15. Fox, C.S., Ramachandran, S., Vasan, M.D. *et al.* (2003) Mitral annular calcification predicts cardiovascular morbidity and mortality. The Framingham Heart Study. *Circulation*, **107**, 1492–1496.

16. Nair, C.K., Thompson, W., Ryschon, K. *et al.* (1989) Long-term follow up of patients with echocardiographically detected mitral annular calcification and comparison with age and sex matched control subjects. *The American Journal of Cardiology*, **63**, 465–470.

17. Aronow, W.S., Ahn, C., Schwartz, K.S. and Koenigsberg, M. (1987) Correlation of atrial fibrillation with presence or absence of mitral annular calcification in 604 subjects older than 60 years. *The American Journal of Cardiology*, **59**, 1213–1214.

18. British Heart Foundation: Coronary Heart Disease statistics, 2006 edition: BHF statistics database. Available at www.heartstats.org.

19. Mosterd, A., Hoes, A.W., de Bruyne, M.C. *et al.* (1999) Prevalence of heart failure and left ventricular dysfunction in the general population. The Rotterdam Study. *European Heart Journal*, **20**, 447–455.

20. Aronow, W.S. (2006) Heart disease and aging. *Medical Clinics of North America*, **90**, 849–862.

21. Kitzman, D., Scholz, D., Hagen, P. *et al.* (1988) Age-related changes in normal human hearts during the first ten decades of life. Part II (Maturity): A quantitative anatomic study of 765 specimens from subjects 20 to 99 years old. *Mayo Clinic Proceedings*, **63**, 137–146.

22. Lakatta, E. (1987) Do hypertension and aging have a similar effect on the myocardium? *Circulation*, **75** (Suppl I), I-69.

23. Dunlap, S.H., Sueta, C.A., Tomasko, L. and Adams, K.F. (1999) Association of body mass, gender and race with heart failure primarily due to hypertension. *Journal of the American College of Cardiology*, **34**, 1602–1608.

24. Lakatta, E.G. (2001) Cardiovascular aging without a clinical diagnosis. *Dialogues in Cardiovascular Medicine*, **6**, 67–91.

25. Oxenham, H. and Sharpe, N. (2003) Cardiovascular aging and the heart. *European Journal of Heart Failure*, **5**, 427–434.

26. Olivetti, G., Melissari, M., Capasso, J.M. *et al.* (1991) Cardiomyopathy of the aging human heart. Myocyte loss and reactive cellular hypertrophy. *Circulation Research*, **68**, 1560–1568.

27. Anversa, P., Palackal, T., Sonnenblick, E.H. *et al.* (1990) Myocyte cell loss and myocyte cellular hyperplasia in the hypertrophied aging rat heart. *Circulation Research*, **67**, 871–885.

28. Lakatta, E. (1993) Cardiovascular regulatory mechanisms in advanced age. *Physiological Reviews*, **73**, 413–467.

29. Ganau, A., Saba, P.S., Roman, M.J. *et al.* (1995) Ageing induces left ventricular concentric remodelling in normotensive subjects. *Journal of Hypertension*, **13**, 1818–1822.

30. Oxenham, H.C., Young, A.A., Cowan, B.R. *et al.* (2003) Age-related changes in myocardial relaxation using three-dimensional tagged magnetic resonance imaging. *Journal of Cardiovascular Magnetic Resonance*, **5** (3), 421–430.

31. Gardin, J.M., Arnold, A.M., Bild, D.E. *et al.* (1998) Left ventricular diastolic filling in the elderly: the cardiovascular health study. *The American Journal of Cardiology*, **82**, 345–351.

32. Sagie, A., Benjamin, E.J., Galderisi, M. *et al.* (1993) Reference values for Doppler indexes of left ventricular diastolic filling in the elderly. *Journal of the American Society of Echocardiography*, **6**, 570–576.

33. Schirmer, H., Lunde, P. and Rasmussen, K. (2000) Mitral flow derived Doppler indices of left ventricular diastolic function in a general population; the Tromso study. *European Heart Journal*, **21**, 1376–1386.

34. Pearson, A., Gudipati, C., Nagelhout, D. *et al.* (1991) Echocardiographic evaluation of cardiac structure and function in elderly subjects with isolated systolic hypertension. *Journal of the American College of Cardiology*, **17**, 422–430.

35. Schoolwerth, A.C., Sica, D.A., Ballerman, B.J. and Wilcox, C.S. (2001) Renal considerations in angiotensin converting enzyme inhibitor therapy: a statement for healthcare professionals from the Council on the Kidney in Cardiovascular Disease and the Council for High Blood Pressure Research of the American Heart Association. *Circulation*, **104**, 1985–1991.

36. Podrazik, P.M. and Schwatz, J.B. (1999) Cardiovascular pharmacology of aging. *Cardiology Clinics: Cardiovascular Disease in the Elderly*, **17**, 17–34.

37. Kottgen, A., Russell, S.D., Loehr, L.R. *et al.* (2007) Reduced kidney function as a risk factor for incident heart failure: The Atherosclerosis Risk in Communities (ARIC) Study. *Journal of the American Society of Nephrology*, **18**, 1307–1315.

38. Gottdiener, J.S., Arnold, A.M., Aurigemma, G.P. *et al.* (2000) Predictors of congestive heart failure in the elderly: the cardiovascular health study. *Journal of the American College of Cardiology*, **35**, 1628–1637.

39. Petrie, M.C. and McMurray, J.J.V. (2007) Dysglycemia and heart failure hospitalisation: what is the link? *Circulation*, **115**, 1334–1335.

40. Libonati, J.R. (1999) Myocardial diastolic function and exercise. *Medicine and Science in Sports and Exercise*, **31**, 1741–1747.

41. Spina, R.J., Turner, M.J. and Ehsani, A.A. (1998) Beta-adrenergic-mediated improvement in left ventricular function by exercise training in older men. *The American Journal of Physiology*, **274**, H397–404.

42. Stratton, J.R., Levy, W.C., Cerqueira, M.D. *et al.* (1994) Cardiovascular responses to exercise. Effects of aging and exercise training in healthy men. *Circulation*, **89**, 1648–1655.

43. Malbut-Shennan, K. and Young, A. (1999) The physiology of physical performance and training in old age. *Coronary Artery Disease*, **10**, 37–42.

44. Rodeheffer, R.J., Gerstenblith, G., Becker, L.C. *et al.* (1984) Exercise cardiac output is maintained with advancing age in healthy human subjects: cardiac dilatation and increased stroke volume compensate for a diminished heart rate. *Circulation*, **69**, 203–213.

45. Friesinger, G.C. and Ryan, T.J. (1999) Coronary artery disease: stable and unstable syndromes. *Cardiology Clinics. Cardiovascular Disease in the Elderly*, **17** (1), 93–122.

46. Ryder, K.M. and Benjamin, E.J. (1999) Epidemiology and significance of atrial fibrillation. *The American Journal of Cardiology*, **84**, 131R–138R.

47. McMurray, J., Komadja, M., Anker, S. and Gardner, R. (2006) Heart failure: epidemiology, pathophysiology and diagnosis, in *The European Society of Cardiology Textbook of Cardiovascular Medicine* (eds J.A. Cramm, T.F. Luscher and P.W. Serryus), Blackwell Publishing, pp. 685–720.

48. Colucci, W.S. and Braunwald, E. (2001) Pathophysiology of heart failure, in *Heart Disease, a Textbook of Cardiovascular Medicine* (eds E. Braunwald, D.P. Zipes and P. Libby), W.B. Saunders Company, pp. 503–533.

49. European Society of Cardiology (2005) HeartScore. Available at www.heartscore.org.

50. Shepherd, J., Blauw, G.J., Murphy, M.B. *et al.* (1999) Prospective study of pravastatin in the elderly at risk. *American Journal of Cardiology*, **84**, 1192–1197.

51. Swinne, C.J., Shapiro, E.P., Lima, S.D. *et al.* (1992) Age-associated changes in left ventricular diastolic performance during isometric exercise in normal subjects. *American Journal of Cardiology*, **69**, 823–826.

52. Tanaka, H., Dinenno, F.A., Monahan, K.D. *et al.* (2000) Aging, habitual exercise, and dynamic arterial compliance. *Circulation*, **102**, 1270–1275.

4

Aetiology

Christopher Ward

Ninewells Hospital and Medical School, Dundee

Key Messages

- Coronary artery disease and hypertension cause 70–80% of cases of heart failure, irrespective of patient age.

- Older patients are more likely to develop heart failure following myocardial infarction than are younger patients.

- Functional mitral regurgitation is the norm in advanced heart failure; it is more common and the prognosis is worse in older patients.

- The aetiology of heart failure dictates the appropriate treatment.

4.1   Classification of the aetiologies of heart failure

Heart failure can be caused by "...any structural or functional cardiac or non cardiac disorder that impairs the ability of the heart to respond to physiological demands for increased cardiac output" [1].

Textbooks and guidelines classify the causes under a series of headings and subheadings, but the similarity ends there. In some books, the major causes are classified anatomically for example as myocardial, valvular (each with several subheadings) and pericardial, with other group headings for the less-common causes [2]; in other books they are classified into pathophysiological groups as

---

A Practical Guide to Heart Failure in Older People, Edited by C Ward and M D Witham
© 2009 John Wiley & Sons, Ltd

Table 4.1 Aetiology of heart failure. (Based on Ref. [2].)

Major categories	Subgroups	Examples
Myocardial disease	Coronary artery disease	
	Hypertension	
	Inflammatory/immune	Viral myocarditis
	Infiltration/metabolic	Amyloidosis
	Endocrine	Thyrotoxicosis
	Toxic	Alcohol
	idiopathic	Dilated cardiomyopathy
Valvular disease		Mitral regurgitation
		Aortic stenosis
Pericardial disease	Effusion	
	constriction	
Endocardial/ endomyocardial disease		
Congenital heart disease		Atrial septal defect
Genetic		Familial cardiomyopathy
Arrhythmias	Tachycardia	Atrial fibrillation
	Bradycardia	Third-degree atrioventricular (A-V) block
High-output states	Anaemia	
	Sepsis	
	Paget's disease	
Volume overload	Renal failure, Iatrogenic	

'underlying', 'fundamental' and 'precipitating' [3] – and there are variations on both of these schemes. This diversity of classifications is confusing, not least because some causes can legitimately be listed under several different headings, even within one classification system [2].

However, in practical terms the differences between the various classifications are of secondary importance – it is more important that the causes are listed rather than listed in a particular way. The information in Table 4.1 is based on the classification used in *The European Society of Cardiology Textbook of Cardiovascular Medicine* [2].

In the developed world, four or five aetiologies are responsible for more than 95% of cases:

- Coronary artery disease (usually myocardial infarction)

- Hypertension, either alone or in combination with coronary artery disease

- Valvular disease, notably mitral regurgitation and aortic stenosis [2]

- The cardiomyopathies

- Atrial fibrillation.

Each of these aetiologies can occur at any time during adult life, but their relative prevalence varies with age. It is also important to appreciate that in older patients, heart failure often results from a combination of pathologies: not only do many people have both coronary artery disease and hypertension, but because of the ubiquity of coronary artery disease with advancing age (see Chapter 3), the majority with valvular disease or a cardiomyopathy will also have concomitant coronary artery diseases. However, identifying the extent to which each pathology is responsible for the patient's condition can be difficult or impossible.

- Hypertension as the primary cause of heart failure is more common in older patients, especially in women [4].

- The prevalence of valvular disease as a cause of heart failure increases with age [5, 6].

- The prevalence of hypertrophic cardiomyopathy also increases with age [7].

4.2   The importance of identifying the aetiology

Identifying the aetiology of heart failure is not an academic exercise:

1. It dictates the most appropriate treatment, and it should therefore be documented as part of the diagnostic process (see Chapter 5).

    - Patients with underlying coronary artery disease should usually be prescribed aspirin, a statin and often also anti-anginal treatment, in addition to the conventional treatment for heart failure.

    - Medication may need to be modified in patients with valvular disease. For example, vasodilating drugs should be avoided or used only with caution in patients with severe aortic stenosis.

    - Selected patients with functional mitral regurgitation, irrespective of its aetiology (see below and Chapter 11), benefit from valvuloplasty and those with coronary artery disease from coronary surgery or angioplasty.

    - Patients with valvular disease should be regarded as potential candidates for appropriate valve surgery on the basis of clinical suitability, not age.

    - The initial treatment for heart failure caused by hypertrophic cardiomyopathy is with a beta-blocker or calcium channel blocker, not an ACE inhibitor [8].

Table 4.2 Factors which affect the reported prevalence of the common causes of heart failure.

The age and gender
The diagnostic criteria used for heart failure and for hypertension
The accuracy of identification of the aetiology
Whether the patient cohort studied was hospital- or community-based
Patient ethnicity
Whether data collection was pre or post the inclusion of patients with HF-PSF.

2. It influences the natural history and prognosis – information to which patients are entitled and which dictates the optimum medication and management:

- In patients with coronary artery disease, hospitalization because of an acute coronary syndrome is common and often leads to further deterioration in left ventricular (LV) function.

- Patients with hypertension or valve disease, who often have HF-PSF (see Chapter 1), have a high incidence of atrial fibrillation which may cause worsening of symptoms and/or embolic complications and require specific additional medication.

- The average life expectancy following the onset of heart failure in patients with aortic stenosis is approximately 18 months (unless they have surgery); this is significantly less than for patients whose heart failure results from coronary artery disease. [9].

The reported prevalence of the different aetiologies varies for a number of reasons (see Table 4.2), most of which can be attributed to the age and gender of the patient cohort studied. For example, hypertension is particularly common in older female patients (see below) – an under-represented group in hospital cohorts which generally include more young male patients.

4.3 Specific aetiologies

Coronary artery disease and hypertension

In developed countries, the majority of cases of heart failure are caused by coronary artery disease and/or hypertension [10]. However, quantifying the percentage of cases caused by one or the other separately, or by a combination of the two, is difficult for several reasons in addition to those noted above:

- In epidemiological studies, the diagnosis of coronary artery disease is usually based on a combination of a documented history of myocardial infarction or

Table 4.3 Heart failure caused by coronary artery disease and/or hypertension (%).

Author	Aetiology identified			Total with each aetiology	
	CAD[a]	BP[b]	CAD + BP	CAD	BP
Cowie et al. [10]	36	44	51	87	95
Wilhelmsen et al. [12]	23.5	20.3	34	57	54

[a]Ref. [10]: includes all acute coronary syndromes, angina and angiographic coronary disease.
[b]BP >165/95 mmHg resting (Ref. [12]); history from GP records or 165/95 mmHg during hospitalization (Ref. [10]).

angina, or by ECG changes showing pathological Q waves or left bundle branch block (as an indication of previous myocardial infarction). However, without coronary angiography, which is less likely to be performed in older patients, other cases will be miss-classified, for example as having hypertensive heart disease or a congestive cardiomyopathy [10].

- If coronary angiography is performed, almost 50% of patients ascribed an alternative diagnosis may prove to have significant underlying coronary artery disease. The same is likely to be true in more than one-third of patients who otherwise would be classified as having no identifiable cause for their heart failure [11]. (This angiographic study excluded patients aged over 75 years in whom the prevalence of unsuspected coronary artery would be expected to be even higher.) Significantly more patients therefore have underlying coronary artery disease than are recorded in epidemiological studies.

- A previously raised blood pressure may be normalized following myocardial infarction, or with the onset of heart failure.

- Many patients are, based on clinical grounds and noninvasive tests, considered to have both coronary artery disease and hypertension (see Table 4.3).

Despite the problems associated with accurately ascribing an aetiology, it is likely that in the region of 80% of cases of heart failure are caused by coronary artery disease and/or hypertension [13] (Figure 4.1).

4.4 Post-myocardial infarction (post-MI) Heart Failure

More than 90% of patients who sustain a myocardial infarction initially have evidence of LV impairment, yet in about one-quarter of these (given optimum reperfusion therapy) normal function will return within 3 months [15].

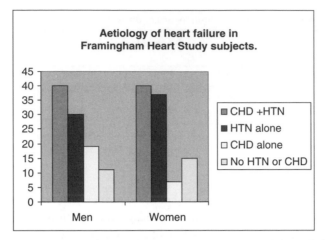

Figure 4.1 Coronary artery disease and hypertension in patients with heart failure. Values are expressed as a percentage of the total number of cases. CHD, coronary heart disease; HTN, hypertension. (Based on data from Ref. [14].) Note: The diagnosis of heart failure was made by noncardiologists and based on clinical findings plus chest X-radiography. A diagnosis of hypertension was defined as 160/95 mmHg or higher, based on the first of three measurements. (Today, neither of these diagnostic criteria would be accepted.)

This topic has been the subject of several detailed reviews, although much of the data quoted has been extracted or extrapolated from studies of selected patients [16–20].

The main conclusions were:

- Myocardial infarction is predominantly a disease of the over-65s [18]. Patients above this age – particularly female patients – are more likely to sustain permanent myocardial damage than those who are younger.

- Some 40% of patients develop new onset of heart failure during the months after myocardial infarction [21], usually because of extensive myocardial damage.

- Subsequently, the incidence of new cases is approximately 3% per year. This is attributed to LV remodelling or myocardial hibernation (or both) [22] in patients in whom the initial myocardial damage was not severe enough to cause heart failure at an earlier stage.

- Some patients who initially have severe LV systolic dysfunction do not develop heart failure [15, 16].

- Not all patients with post-MI heart failure have LV systolic dysfunction, as was previously thought: in fact, 30% have HF-PSF that is probably caused by recurrent episodes of silent ischaemia resulting in a patchy myocardial fibrosis and/or a hibernating myocardium, and not due to coexisting hypertension, as had been assumed [16].

- The mortality from post-MI heart failure increases with age.

4.5 Valvular disease

Mitral regurgitation

More than 90% of patients with heart failure have at least mild mitral regurgitation (MR) [9]:

- MR may cause, or be caused by, heart failure.

- In either case it has a negative impact on the prognosis, even if it is only mild.

- Irrespective of aetiology, the prevalence of MR increases with age. Patients with severe post-MI MR (see below) are on average 10 years older than those with no MR [23].

- Myocardial infarction, being the major cause of heart failure, is likewise the commonest cause of MR.

The causes of MR are usually divided into: (i) those which are functional – that is, not the result of valvular pathology; and (ii) those caused by valvular disease. Of these two, functional MR is by far the largest in terms of patient numbers (Table 4.4).

Mitral regurgitation caused by left ventricular dilatation (functional MR)

Functional MR is a consequence of the LV dilatation that occurs during the development of heart failure (LV remodelling). This process alters the shape of the ventricle from its normal elliptical form to one which is more globular and dilated. This results in a misalignment of the papillary muscles so that coaptation of the valve cusps during systole – which is essential to prevent MR – is no longer possible. This occurs in association with heart failure, irrespective of aetiology. Coronary artery

Table 4.4 Causes of mitral regurgitation in older patients. (Based on data from Ref. [24]).

Functional MR: Left ventricular dilatation from any cause. Usually myocardial infarction
Post-MI papillary muscle rupture/ischaemia
Mitral annular calcification
Mitral valve prolapse (myxomatous valve degeneration)

disease (notably myocardial infarction), in being the major cause of heart failure, is the commonest underlying pathology.

Functional MR is, by definition, a consequence of heart failure and therefore not a cause. It has nevertheless been included in this chapter as it consistently leads to a worsening of heart failure symptoms and prognosis. For these reasons, it should be actively sought and its presence routinely documented as a part of the risk assessment/stratification of all heart failure patients.

The prevalence of functional MR increases in line with the progression of LV dilatation and with a deterioration in functional status. Approximately 90% of patients with advanced heart failure (NYHA class III or IV) have MR, and in 40% of these it is deemed to be moderate or severe [25, 26]. Those patients with the most severe MR have a poorer functional capacity and a worse prognosis [25], although even in these cases there is often no audible murmur. Echocardiography is therefore essential in order to determine the severity of MR and hence the patient's risk profile [25, 27].

Post-infarction mitral regurgitation

- MR can be detected in 50% of patients within a few days of MI. In almost 40% of cases it is mild, while in 10% it is moderate/severe [23, 26, 28].

- In approximately 1% of cases the MR is caused by infarction of a papillary muscle, causing the muscle to rupture [29].

- Other than in this small group, MR is functional and the result of LV impairment, as discussed above. Usually, LV systolic dysfunction is present, but in some patients the LV function is preserved (i.e. in HF-PSF).

- The prevalence and severity of post-infarction MR, and therefore of heart failure [26], increases with a history of previous infarction, the extent of myocardial damage, older age and female gender [26, 28].

- Over 60% of patients who initially have moderate/severe post-MI MR and who survive for 5 years have heart failure; the same is true of almost 40% of those with only mild MR [28].

- There is no audible murmur in the majority of patients with post-infarction MR.

- Left atrial enlargement, LV enlargement and pulmonary congestion are more pronounced when MR results from MI than when it is valvular [28]. This is because, in the latter situation, the LV contractility is initially normal and can increase to compensate for the valve defect. This is not possible with functional MR because the ventricle is already impaired as a result of the infarction.

Mitral annular calcification (MAC)

MAC is a degenerative process in which calcium is deposited crescentically around the base of the mitral valve. This impedes normal valve closure, thus causing MR. The condition is uncommon before the age of 50 [30], but subsequently the prevalence of each stage in the progression from MAC via MR to heart failure is age-related:

- The prevalence of MAC rises from 20% at the age of 60–65 to more than 60% in the over-80s (see Figure 4.2).

- Some 20–33% of patients with MAC have moderate to severe MR.

- Up to 40% of patients develop heart failure within a few years of the identification of MAC [30].

- In addition to causing MR, MAC is associated with conventional cardiovascular risk factors, and therefore with an increased prevalence of myocardial infarction, angina and cardiovascular-related mortality [31].

Mitral valve prolapse and myxomatous degeneration of the mitral valve

Mitral valve prolapse (MVP) is characterized anatomically by an increase in the area of the thickened valve leaflets. It is associated with specific auscultatory and echocardiographic findings [33], and was initially considered to be a common quite benign condition which affected predominantly young women. In this case the

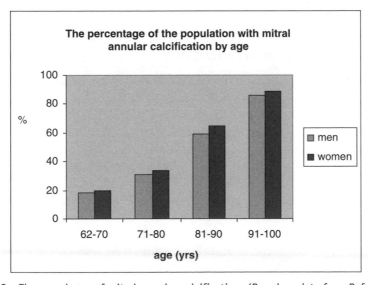

Figure 4.2 The prevalence of mitral annular calcification. (Based on data from Ref. [32].)

condition was referred to as MVP syndrome. There exists, however, a second group of predominantly older men in whom MVP is associated with myxomatous degeneration of the valve cusps, a high incidence of rupture of the chordae tendineae, and with a significant risk of progressing from MVP to severe MR and heart failure over a number of years [34]. However, because of the clinical overlap between these groups, and a lack of agreement about the precise echocardiographic criteria, very limited reliable data are available on the epidemiology and natural history of MVP [35].

- Myxomatous degeneration of the mitral valve has been found in 5% of routine post-mortem examinations [36].

- In the same study, one-half of the patients with myxomatous degeneration of the mitral valve had suffered heart failure.

- This is consistent with the finding that one-half of symptomatic patients with MVP aged over 60 years have heart failure [34].

- The risk of patients with MVP developing severe MR increases after the age of 50 [37].

  - Most patients with heart failure have MR.

  - It is usually functional, the result of extensive LV damage or remodelling, and occurs irrespective of the aetiology.

  - Functional MR is more common in older patients, and has a major impact on the progression and prognosis of heart failure.

  - Clinical examination fails to identify MR in the majority of cases; echocardiography is essential for its detection.

  - The presence and severity of MR should always be documented.

Aortic sclerosis and aortic stenosis

Degenerative calcific aortic stenosis is the commonest valve lesion in older patients [38].

Although aortic stenosis is an uncommon cause of heart failure when compared to coronary artery disease, it is important because timely surgery can be effectively curative, even in patients of advanced age (see Chapter 11).

A number of studies in recent years have reported an association between aortic sclerosis (thickening of the aortic valve cusps without obstruction; TAV) and both conventional cardiovascular risk factors and age [39] (as is the case with MAC; see

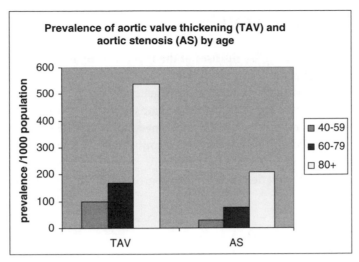

Figure 4.3 Aortic stenosis: defined as peak systolic gradient ≥20 mmHg. (Based on data from Ref. [43].)

above). Moreover, as TAV is the precursor of aortic stenosis these studies may also explain the age-related increase in the prevalence of the latter condition, and of its frequent coexistence with coronary artery disease.

The prevalence of TAV doubles between the ages of 20 and 65 years [40], and subsequently increases from 25% between the ages of 65 and 74 years to 48% in those aged over 75 [38] (Figure 4.3). The prevalence of aortic valve calcification more or less parallels that of aortic sclerosis, being present in more than 50% of subjects aged 75–86 years. The end result is that between 2% and 18% of the older subjects have some degree of aortic stenosis, usually defined as an aortic valve gradient of greater than 20–25 mmHg [39, 41]. The higher figure, confined to patients all aged over 80 years, identified the stenosis as severe (2%), moderate (6%) and mild (10%) [42].

The average age at which symptoms of aortic stenosis develop is 70–80 years [39], and in this age group almost 50% of patients with severe stenosis will eventually develop heart failure [9].

Based on the results of two general practice studies conducted in England [44, 45], the prevalence of aortic stenosis as the primary cause of heart failure was seen to be 6–9%, and was almost twice as common in the over-75s than in younger patients [46].

Because of the high prevalence of overt and subclinical coronary artery disease in older patients with aortic stenosis (approximately 50% have significant coronary artery disease) [39, 46], it is inevitable that many cases will be of mixed aetiology.

4.6   The cardiomyopathies

The cardiomyopathies are ". . .diseases of the myocardium associated with cardiac dysfunction" [47], but excluding those cases caused by inflammatory diseases (which are classed as myocarditis). The diagnosis is generally described as a 'diagnosis by exclusion', as it is reserved for those conditions affecting the myocardium after coronary artery, hypertensive, valvular and congenital heart disease have been ruled out [48]. The latter conditions have however, confusingly, been officially classified as specific cardiomyopathies [47].

In routine clinical practice three main subgroups of the cardiomyopathies are usually described:

- Dilated cardiomyopathies

- Hypertrophic cardiomyopathy (HCM)

- Restrictive cardiomyopathies.

There are several other classifications of the many causes of the cardiomyopathies, detailed accounts of which are provided in standard textbooks [48, 49].

The cardiomyopathies, taken together, cause perhaps 10–20% of all cases of heart failure in which there is LV systolic dysfunction [2], but because approximately one-half of patients have HF-PSF (see Chapter 2) the overall prevalence is nearer to 5–10%. With the possible exception of HCM, cardiomyopathies are less common in older patients [6, 7].

The treatment of most patients with a cardiomyopathy is currently the same as that for most other cases of heart failure. In practice, irrespective of the patient's age, there is rarely a serious attempt made to identify if they have a cardiomyopathy – and certainly not to establish which of the many possible causes is responsible. For these various reasons the topic is discussed only briefly here. Having said that, patients suspected of having hypertrophic or restrictive cardiomyopathy should be referred for specialist advice.

Hypertrophic cardiomyopathy (HCM)

In early reports, HCM (previously known as hypertrophic obstructive cardiomyop-athy; HOCM) was considered to be predominantly a disease of the young and middle-aged, but this is clearly not the case. A number of studies conducted during the past 20 years have reported that one-third or more of patients are aged over 65 years, a majority of whom are female – in contrast to the male preponderance in younger patients [8, 50, 51]. Previously, cases in older patients were often overlooked for two reasons:

- Clinically, prior to the widespread use of echocardiography, patients were incorrectly diagnosed as having coronary artery disease, hypertension or aortic stenosis [51].

- There is a group of mainly (80%) older female patients who have established hypertension and gross left ventricular hypertrophy (LVH). These patients have previously been described as having hypertensive hypertrophic cardiomyopathy and classified as a subgroup of HCM [52].

However, this is misleading as the natural history, epidemiology and histological findings of this condition are distinct from those of HCM. Such patients are now considered to have an extreme expression of the LVH normally present in hypertension and not a specific cardiomyopathy, nor a variant of HCM [53].

Over a three-year period, between 10 and 20% of older patients with HCM develop a clinical picture typical of a congestive cardiomyopathy [54], but the figure (for all age groups) rises to 60% if they have previously had severe LVH [55].

There are important reasons for identifying patients with HCM; the recommended initial treatment is with a beta-blocker or a calcium channel blocker such as verapamil rather than with an ACE inhibitor [8]. Also, when the diagnosis is confirmed, family members should be screened as most cases are inherited on an autosomal dominant basis.

Restrictive cardiomyopathy

Amyloidosis is often quoted as a cause of restrictive cardiomyopathy in older patients but is rare; on the other hand, amyloid deposits are a quite common incidental finding in the hearts of the very old [6].

However, if this or any other restrictive cardiomyopathy is suspected on the basis of echocardiography, the patient should be referred to a cardiologist: aetiology-specific treatment may be appropriate and the screening of family members may be advisable.

4.7 Atrial fibrillation

Atrial fibrillation is common in heart failure, being present in almost one-third of newly diagnosed cases; moreover, the prevalence increases with age. Although atrial fibrillation is often described as a comorbidity of heart failure, in approximately 5% of cases it is now considered to be the cause [11]. Heart failure symptoms often improve as a result of rate control or a return to sinus rhythm, and in a few cases it is cured. Usually, however, it is impossible to decide whether atrial fibrillation is the cause or a result of heart failure.

References

1. Scottish Intercollegiate Guidelines Network (SIGN 95) (2007) Management of Chronic Heart Failure. A National Clinical Guideline. Royal College of Physicians, Edinburgh. Available at www.sign.ac.uk.
2. McMurray, J., Komadja, M., Anker, S. and Gardner, R. (2006) Heart failure: epidemiology, pathophysiology and diagnosis, in *The European Society of Cardiology Textbook of Cardiovascular Medicine* (eds J.A. Cramm, T.F. Luscher and P.W. Serryus), Blackwell Publishing, pp. 685–720.
3. Givertz, M.M., Colucci, W.S. and Braunwald, E. (2001) Clinical aspects of heart failure, in *Heart Disease, A Textbook of Cardiovascular Medicine*, 6th edn (eds E. Braunwald, D.P. Zipes and P. Libby), Chapter 17, W.B. Saunders Company.
4. Owan, T.E. and Redfield, M.M. (2005) Epidemiology of diastolic heart failure. *Progress in Cardiovascular Disease*, **47** (5), 320–332.
5. Rahimatojola, S.H., Cheitlin, M.D. and Hutter, M.M. (1987) Valvular and congenital heart disease. *Journal of the American College of Cardiology*, **10** (Suppl A), 60A–62A.
6. Rich, M.W. (1999) Heart failure. *Cardiology Clinics*, **17** (1), 123–135.
7. Shah, P.M., Abelmann, W.H. and Gersh, B.J. (1987) Cardiomyopathies in the elderly. *Journal of the American College of Cardiology*, **10** (A), 77A–79A.
8. Marron, B.J. (1997) Hypertrophic cardiomyopathy. *The Lancet*, **350**, 127–133.
9. Varadarajan, P., Kapoor, N., Bansal, R.C. *et al.* (2006) Clinical profile and natural history of 543 patients non surgically managed with severe aortic stenosis. *Annals of Thoracic Surgery*, **82**, 2111–2115.
10. Cowie, M.R., Wood, D.A., Coats, A.J.S. *et al.* (1999) Incidence and aetiology of heart failure: a population-based study. *European Heart Journal*, **20**, 421–428.
11. Fox, K.F., Cowie, M.R., Wood, D.A. *et al.* (2001) Coronary artery disease as the cause of incident heart failure in the population. *European Heart Journal*, **22**, 228–236.
12. Wilhelmsen, L., Rosengren, A., Eriksson, H. *et al.* (2001) Heart failure in the general population – morbidity, risk factors and prognosis. *Journal of Internal Medicine*, **249**, 253–261.
13. Gheorghaide, M. and Bonow, R. (1998) Chronic heart failure in the United States: a manifestation of coronary artery disease. *Circulation*, **97** (3), 282–289.
14. Kannel, W.B. (1997) Epidemiology of heart failure in the United States, in *Heart Failure* (eds P.A. Poole-Wilson, W.S. Colucci and B.M. Massie *et al.*), Ch. 20, Churchill Livingstone, pp. 279–288.
15. Solomon, S.D., Glynn, R.J., Greaves, S. *et al.* (2001) Recovery of ventricular function after myocardial infarction in the reperfusion era: the healing and early afterload reducing therapy study. *Annals of Internal Medicine*, **134**, 451–458.
16. Cleland, J.G.F., Torabi, A. and Khan, N.K. (2005) Epidemiology and management of heart failure and left ventricular systolic dysfunction in the aftermath of a myocardial infarction. *Heart*, **9** (Suppl II), ii7–ii13.
17. Hellermann, J.P., Jacobsen, S.J., Redfield, M.M. *et al.* (2005) Heart failure after myocardial infarction: clinical presentation and survival. *European Journal of Heart Failure*, **7**, 119–125.

18. Friesinger, G.C. and Ryan, T.J. (1999) Coronary heart disease: Stable and unstable syndromes. *Cardiology Clinics: Cardiovascular Disease in the Elderly*, **17** (1), 93–122.

19. Hellermann, J.P., Jacobsen, S.J., Reeder, G.S. *et al.* (2003) Heart failure after myocardial infarction: relevance of preserved left ventricular systolic function in the community. *American Heart Journal*, **145**, 742–748.

20. Hellermann, J.P., Jacobsen, S.J., Gersh, B.J. *et al.* (2002) Heart failure after myocardial infarction: a review. *American Journal of Medicine*, **113**, 324–330.

21. Ali, A.S., Rybicki, B.A., Aslam, M. *et al.* (1999) Clinical predictors of heart failure in patients with first myocardial infarction. *American Heart Journal*, **138** (6), 1133–1139.

22. Fox, K.F., Cowie, M.R., Wood, D.A. *et al.* (1999) New perspectives on heart failure due to myocardial ischaemia. *European Heart Journal*, **20**, 256–262.

23. Bursi, F., Enriquez-Sarano, M., Nkomo, V.T. *et al.* (2005) Heart failure and death after myocardial infarction in the community: the emerging role of mitral regurgitation. *Circulation*, **111**, 295–301.

24. Cheitlin, M.D. and Aronow, W.S. (2004) Mitral regurgitation, mitral stenosis and mitral annular calcification in the elderly, in *Cardiovascular Disease in the Elderly*, 3rd edn (eds W.S. Aronow and J.L. Fleg), Marcel Dekker, New York, pp. 443–476.

25. Patel, J.B., Borgeson, D.D., Barnes, M.E. *et al.* (2004) Mitral regurgitation in patients with advanced systolic heart failure. *Journal of Cardiac Failure*, **10** (4), 2285–2291.

26. Aronson, D., Goldsher, N., Zuckermann, R. *et al.* (2006) Ischaemic mitral regurgitation and risk of heart failure after myocardial infarction. *Archives of Internal Medicine*, **166**, 2362–2368.

27. Varadarajan, P., Sharma, S., Heywood, T. *et al.* (2006) High prevalence of clinically silent severe mitral regurgitation in patients with heart failure: role for echocardiography. *Journal of the American Society of Echocardiography*, **19**, 1458–1461.

28. Bursi, F., Enriquez-Sarano, M., Jacobsen, S.J. *et al.* (2006) Mitral regurgitation after myocardial infarction: a review. *The American Journal of Medicine*, **119**, 103–112.

29. Sharma, S.M., Secklerr, J., Israel, D.H. *et al.* (1992) Angiographic and anatomic findings in acute severe ischaemic mitral regurgitation. *The American Journal of Cardiology*, **70**, 277–280.

30. Nair, C.K., Thompson, W., Ryschon, K. *et al.* (1989) Long term follow-up of patients with echocardiographically detected mitral annular calcium and comparison with age-and-sex matched control subjects. *The American Journal of Cardiology*, **63**, 465–470.

31. Barasch, J., Gottdiener, J.S., Larsen, E.K. *et al.* (2006) Cardiovascular morbidity and mortality in community-dwelling elderly individuals with calcification of the fibrous skeleton at the base of the heart and aortosclerosis (The Cardiovascular Health Study). *The American Journal of Cardiology*, **97**, 1281–1286.

32. Aronow, W.S., Schwartz, K.S. and Koenigsberg, M. (1987) Correlation of atrial fibrillation with presence or absence of mitral annular calcification in 604 persons older than 60 years. *The American Journal of Cardiology*, **59**, 1213–1214.

33. Perloff, J.K., Child, J.S. and Edwards, J.E. (1986) New guidelines for the clinical diagnosis of mitral valve prolapse. *The American Journal of Cardiology*, **57**, 1124–1129.

34. Kolibash, A.J., Bush, C.A., Fontana, M.B. *et al.* (1983) Mitral valve prolapse syndrome: analysis of 62 patients aged 62 years and older. *The American Journal of Cardiology*, **52**, 534–539.

35. Otto, C.M. (1999) Mitral valve prolapse, in *Valvular Heart Disease* (ed. C.M. Otto), W.B. Saunders Company, Ch. 14, pp. 323–339.

36. Pomerance, A. (1969) Ballooning deformity (mucoid degeneration) of atrioventricular valves. *British Heart Journal*, **31**, 343–351.

37. Wilken, D.E.L. and Hickey, A.J. (1988) Lifetime risk for patients with mitral valve prolapse of developing severe valve regurgitation requiring surgery. *Circulation*, **78**, 10–14.

38. Hinchman, D.A. and Otto, C.M. (1999) Valvular disease in the elderly. *Cardiology Clinics: Cardiovascular Disease in the Elderly*, **17**, 137–158.

39. Otto, C.M., Lind, B.K., Kitzman, D.W. *et al.* (1999) Association of aortic valve sclerosis with cardiovascular mortality and morbidity in the elderly. *The New England Journal of Medicine*, **341**, 142–147.

40. Sahasakul, Y., Edwards, W.D., Naessens, J.M. *et al.* (1988) Age-related changes in aortic and mitral valve thickness: implications for two-dimensional echocardiography based on an autopsy study of 200 normal human hearts. *The American Journal of Cardiology*, **62**, 4224–4230.

41. Stewart, B.F., Siskovick, D., Lind, B.K. *et al.* (1997) Clinical factors associated with calcific aortic valve disease: cardiovascular health study. *Journal of the American College of Cardiology*, **29**, 630–634.

42. Aronow, W.S. and Kronzon, I. (1991) Prevalence and severity of valvular aortic stenosis determined by doppler echocardiography and its association with echocardiographic and electrocardiographic left ventricular hypertrophy and physical signs of aortic stenosis in elderly patients. *The American Journal of Cardiology*, **67**, 776–777.

43. Lin, S.-L., Liu, C.-P., Young, S.-T. *et al.* (2005) Age-related changes in aortic valve with emphasis on the relation between pressure loading and thickened leaflets of the aortic valve. *International Journal of Cardiology*, **103**, 272–279.

44. Paramashwar, J., Shackell, M.M., Richardson, A. *et al.* (1992) Prevalence of heart failure in three general practices in north west London. *British Journal of General Practice*, **42**, 487–489.

45. Mair, F.S., Crowley, T.S. and Bundred, P.E. (1996) Prevalence, aetiology and management of heart failure in general practice. *British Journal of General Practice*, **46**, 77–79.

46. Silaruks, S., Clark, D., Thinkhamrop, B. *et al.* (2001) Angina pectoris and coronary artery disease in severe isolated valvular aortic stenosis. *Heart Lung and Circulation*, **10**, 14–23.

47. Richardson, P., McKenna, W., Bristow, M. *et al.* (1996) Report of the 1995 World Health Organization/International Society and Federation Task Force on the Definition and Classification of Cardiomyopathies. *Circulation*, **93**, 841–842.

48. Wynne, J. and Braunwald, E. (2001) The cardiomyopathies and myocarditidies, in *Heart Disease, A Textbook of Cardiovascular Medicine*, 6th edn (eds E. Braunwald, D.P. Zipes and P. Libby), W.B. Saunders Company, pp. 1751–1806.

49. Hess, O.M., McKenna, W., Schultheiss, H.-P. *et al.* (2006) Myocardial disease, in *The European Society of Cardiology Textbook of Cardiovascular Medicine* (eds J.A. Cramm, T.F. Luscher and P.W. Serryus), Blackwell Publishing, Ch. 16, pp. 453–515.

50. Cannan, C.R., Reeder, G.S., Bailey, K.R. *et al.* (1995) Natural history of hypertrophic cardiomyopathy: a population-based study, 1976 through 1990. *Circulation*, **92**, 2488–2495.

51. Krasnow, M. and Stein, R.A. (1978) Hypertrophic cardiomyopathy in the aged. *American Heart Journal*, **96**, 326–336.

52. Topol, E.J., Traill, T.A. and Fortuin, N.J. (1985) Hypertensive hypertrophic cardiomyopathy of the elderly. *New England Journal of Medicine*, **312**, 277–283.

53. Roelandt, J. and Erbel, R. (2006) Cardiac ultrasound, in *The European Society of Cardiology Textbook of Cardiovascular Medicine* (eds J.A. Cramm, T.F. Luscher and P.W. Serryus), Blackwell Publishing, Ch. 2, pp. 37–93.

54. Spirito, P., Maron, B.J., Bonow, R.O. *et al.* (1987) Occurrence and significance of progressive left ventricular wall thinning and relative cavity dilatation in hypertrophic cardiomyopathy. *American Journal of Cardiology*, **59**, 123–129.

55. Thaman, R., Gimeno, J.R., Reith, S. *et al.* (2004) Progressive left ventricular remodelling in patients with hypertrophic cardiomyopathy and severe left ventricular hypertrophy. *Journal of the American College of Cardiology*, **44**, 398–405.

5
Diagnosis

Christopher Ward

Ninewells Hospital and Medical School, Dundee

Key messages

- A diagnosis of heart failure based only on the history and clinical findings is usually incorrect.

- An ECG ± a B-type natriuretic peptide (BNP) assay should be requested in all suspected cases: echocardiography should be performed if either test is abnormal.

- In approximately 50% of cases – mostly older patients – left ventricular systolic function is normal or only mildly impaired.

- A high index of suspicion is necessary to identify heart failure in older patients because atypical signs and symptoms are common.

- A diagnosis of heart failure should always be considered in the context of the patient's comorbidities and clinical profile.

There are widely publicised international, national and local guidelines to aid the accurate and prompt diagnosis of heart failure. Yet, often in patients who later prove to have heart failure the initial diagnosis is incorrect, delayed or incomplete. This is particularly common in older patients. A number of factors have been identified which contribute to this, and these will be discussed in the following sections.

A Practical Guide to Heart Failure in Older People, Edited by C Ward and M D Witham
© 2009 John Wiley & Sons, Ltd

5.1   Diagnostic guidelines

Guidelines for the diagnosis and management of chronic heart failure have been published by the European Society of Cardiology (ESC) [1], the American Heart Association/American College of Cardiology (AHA/ACC) [2] and the Scottish Intercollegiate Guidelines Network (SIGN) [3]. Although these guidelines are recommended as the basis for diagnosis in all age groups, they do not address the prevalent atypical mode of presentation of many older patients.

The ESC criteria [1] are concise and unequivocal:

Essential features:

- Symptoms of heart failure at rest or during exercise (e.g. breathlessness, fatigue, ankle swelling) and objective evidence of cardiac dysfunction (systolic and/or diastolic) at rest, preferably by echocardiography.

Non-essential features:

- In cases where the diagnosis is in doubt, there is a response to treatment directed towards heart failure.

The recommendations of the AHA/ACC and SIGN guidelines [2, 3] are similar but are presented in a stepwise clinical approach:

- 'Heart failure (HF) is defined as a clinical syndrome that is characterized by specific symptoms (dyspnoea and fatigue) in the medical history and signs (oedema, rales) on the physical examination. There is no single diagnostic test for HF because it is largely a clinical diagnosis that is based on a careful history and physical examination.

- Two-dimensional echocardiography with Doppler should be performed during an initial evaluation of patients presenting with heart failure to assess left ventricular ejection fraction (LVEF), left ventricular (LV) size, wall thickness and valve function' [2].

Each set of guidelines therefore, bases the diagnostic process on two principles. First, the patient should have a combination of typical symptoms and signs. Second, there should be objective evidence of LV dysfunction. Implicit in the criteria is that patients with heart failure are symptomatic, but that symptoms alone are insufficient to firmly establish the diagnosis.

The requirement for objective evidence of LV dysfunction is because the signs and symptoms of heart failure, irrespective of patient's age, are insensitive and/or nonspecific. As a result, if used in isolation many patients will be misdiagnosed, some will be erroneously treated for heart failure, while in others the diagnosis may be overlooked. These pitfalls are more common in older patients (see below.)

5.2 Symptoms and signs: sensitivity and specificity

An understanding of the implication of these terms is central to appreciating the basis for the difficulty in making a clinical diagnosis of heart failure:

- The sensitivity of a symptom or sign is the percentage of patients (with heart failure) in whom the symptom/sign is identified. (The low sensitivity of a clinical sign does not necessarily mean that it is absent; it may be present but not sought or detected by the examiner.)

- Specificity is the percentage of patients who do not have heart failure and in whom the symptom/sign is absent or negative.

Ideally, the sensitivity and specificity of a symptom or sign would be 100% – that is, it would be easily identified in all patients with the condition, and in nobody else (Table 5.1).

As noted above, an important cause of the poor sensitivity of the signs of heart failure is that, although present, the examining doctor may fail to detect them. However, it is also important to note that several of the classical findings in heart failure – radiological evidence of cardiomegaly, basal crepitations, peripheral oedema and an elevated venous pressure – are often genuinely absent.

- A third of patients with unequivocal heart failure have a normal-sized heart on chest X-ray [4].

- Basal crepitations (rales) indicate heart failure of rapid onset but are absent in most patients with chronic heart failure, even when it is severe and resistant to treatment. This is because in chronic heart failure interstitial fluid is removed by increased lymphatic drainage [5].

- Studies using I^{131} tagged albumin have shown that peripheral oedema is absent in at least half of patients with intravascular fluid overload [6].

- An elevated jugular venous pressure is only observed when the right atrial pressure exceeds a critical value, and this often does not occur [5].

Table 5.1 The implications of poor sensitivity and specificity of symptoms and signs.

Symptoms

Dyspnoea	Dyspnoea occurs in 2/3 heart failure patients,
Orthopnoea	but also in 1/2 of non-heart failure patients;
Paroxysmal nocturnal dyspnoea	the other symptoms occur in less than 1/3 of
History of oedema	heart failure patients and in 1/5 of other
	patients.

Signs

Raised jugular venous pressure	A third heart sound is detected in 1/3 of cases.
Third heart sound	None of the other signs is identified in more
Peripheral oedema, tachycardia,	than 1/8 cases.
crepitations	

Based on data from Ref. [3].

5.3 Objective evidence of left ventricular systolic dysfunction

The diagnostic problems caused by the lack of reliability of clinical findings highlight the need for an objective confirmatory test.

Echocardiography

Transthoracic Doppler echocardiography is the key confirmatory investigation and, in conjunction with the clinical history and examination, will in most cases also point to the aetiology.

The AHA/ACC guidelines list the questions to which echocardiography can provide answers:

- Is the structure of the left ventricle normal or abnormal?

- Is the LVEF preserved or reduced? (see below).

- Is there evidence of LV hypertrophy?

- Are there other structural abnormalities such as valvular, pericardial or right ventricular abnormalities that could account for the clinical presentation?

The most useful measurement for the confirmation of LV systolic dysfunction (HF-LVSD) is the LVEF. This is usually considered to be reduced if it is less than 40% (0.40) and 'preserved' if greater than 50% (0.50), although many patients with HF-PSF fall into the grey area (LVEF 40–50%) between the two. Despite the importance placed on these figures, echocardiography is a relatively inaccurate means of measuring the LVEF when compared to other methods [7] (see below). Unfortunately, these alternative methods have a number of drawbacks.

Other imaging techniques

Cardiac magnetic resonance (CMR) provides the most comprehensive assessment of cardiac structures, size and function [7], and can in some instances identify specific cardiomyopathies such as amyloidosis [8]; however, it is an expensive investigative technique with very limited access.

Radionuclide angiography can be used to assess ventricular size and function. The results are more reproducible than with echocardiography, but it provides no information about valvular function.

Although echocardiography has limitations with respect to reproducibility and diagnostic precision compared to these alternative imaging techniques, it has the overriding practical advantages of lower cost, flexibility in use (portability of equipment) and easy accessibility.

The diagnosis of heart failure with preserved left ventricular function (HF-PSF) (see also Chapter 2)

- In approximately 50% of cases of heart failure, LV systolic function is normal or only mildly reduced (HF-PSF), the problem being an abnormality of diastolic (not systolic) function.

- Patients with HF-PSF are older than those with HF-LVSD, and the majority are female; this gender difference increases with advancing age (see Chapter 2).

- Confirming a diagnosis of HF-PSF is less clear-cut than in HF-LVSD because of the technical and logistical difficulties (see below) in demonstrating relevant echocardiographic abnormalities.

Despite these differences and difficulties, the ESC and AHA/ACC guidelines [1, 2] agree that the diagnosis of HF-PSF should, as with HF-LVSD, be based on a combination of signs and/or symptoms of heart failure plus evidence of ventricular dysfunction, but in the case of HF-PSF, of abnormal *diastolic* function.

The ESC guidelines [1] require the following criteria to be fulfilled to confirm the diagnosis:

- Signs and symptoms of heart failure

- A normal or near-normal LVEF (40–50%)

- Evidence of abnormal LV relaxation, diastolic distensibility or diastolic stiffness (each of these features being a marker of abnormal diastolic function).

It is the documentation of these echocardiographic criteria which is problematic:

- There is no agreed 'best way' to measure these parameters, nor a consensus on which is the most useful (in fact, they may even vary in an individual patient, depending on their haemodynamic status at the time of the examination).

- Some measurements are invasive.

- Many departments lack the equipment and/or expertise to assess diastolic function [1].

These difficulties are acknowledged in the pragmatic approach to the dilemma suggested in the AHA/ACC guidelines [2]:

> "*In practice, the diagnosis of HF-PSF is generally based on the finding of typical symptoms and signs of HF in a patient who is shown to have a normal LVEF... on echocardiography*".... but "every effort should be made to exclude other possible explanations or disorders that may present in a similar manner." (i.e. other explanations for the normal LVEF.)

Alternative explanations to HF-PSF in patients with a clinical diagnosis of heart failure and echocardiographic findings of a normal ejection fraction include (based on Ref. [9]):

- A delay in performing echocardiography in patients with effectively treated HF-LVSD (e.g. episodic severe myocardial ischaemia, tachycardia induced transient pulmonary oedema) or severe hypertension

- Isolated right heart failure (e.g. pulmonary hypertension, right ventricular infarction, cor pulmonale)

- Constrictive pericarditis or effusion

- High-output cardiac failure

- Obesity

- Normal aging (see Chapter 3).

However this does not address the problem of diagnosing HF-PSF in older patients, many of whom lack 'typical symptoms and signs of HF' (see below).

In this situation, HF-PSF should be suspected if a patient has:

- Alternative presenting signs or symptoms known to occur in older patients (see below).

- An abnormal ECG or raised level of BNP or N-terminal pro-BNP (NT pro-BNP).

- Echocardiographic evidence of a normal or near-normal LVEF ± left ventricular hypertrophy.

Many such patients will fit into one the following groups:

- The typical patient with HF-PSF is female and hypertensive, or has a history of hypertension; they are also more likely to have diabetes and/or atrial fibrillation than patients with HF-LVSD.

- There is a history or evidence of one of the other recognized causes of HF-PSF, namely coronary artery disease, aortic stenosis or hypertrophic cardiomyopathy.

'Rule-out' investigations: the role of electrocardiography and brain natriuretic peptides (BNPs)

Although guidelines stress that the diagnosis of heart failure is unsafe without objective evidence of LV dysfunction, this does not mean that all patients in whom the diagnosis is suspected on clinical grounds should undergo echocardiography. Many can be ruled out by using simpler and cheaper tests.

The SIGN guideline [3] advises that: "BNP or NT pro-BNP levels and/or an ECG should be recorded to indicate the need for echocardiography in patients with suspected heart failure". The plasma levels of BNP and NT pro-BNP are raised in both HF-LVSD and HF-PSF [10]. Consequently, unless one or the other of the tests (BNP or ECG) is abnormal, it is very unlikely that the patient has heart failure, and consequently echocardiography would be unnecessary. These are therefore 'rule-out' tests only. In the case of BNP, this is because there are several causes other than heart failure for a raised plasma level, including female gender, advancing age, renal dysfunction, pulmonary embolism, LV hypertrophy and hypertension [7]. Likewise, many people have an abnormal ECG without having heart failure.

The diagnostic strategy in the SIGN guideline [3] is not only more cost-effective than the routine screening of all patients with suspicious symptoms and/or signs by echocardiography, but will also often avoid the difficulties associated with trying to organize hospital visits for frail (or reluctant) older patients in order for them to undergo investigations.

However, because a raised plasma level of BNP does not 'rule in' a diagnosis of heart failure, it is likely that there will always be some frail older patients who, for understandable practical reasons, will continue to be managed on the basis of signs and symptoms alone, without objective evidence that they have LV dysfunction (Figure 5.1).

5.4   Diagnostic difficulties in older patients

Diagnostic guidelines and older patients

The difficulties of diagnosing heart failure, as discussed above, are compounded in older patients for a variety of reasons:

- The symptoms and signs of heart failure listed in published guidelines are based predominantly on findings in relatively young hospitalized patients, the majority of whom presented with acute severe cardiac decompensation [5].

- In contrast, most community-based patients are older, are chronically ill, and have relatively mild symptoms [11]. The classical symptoms and signs, which are integral to the recommended diagnostic process, occur less often in these older patients [12–14] (see below).

- Not only are clinical findings in older patients atypical, but for a combination of practical, financial and administrative reasons the requirement for echocardio-graphic evidence of LV dysfunction to confirm the diagnosis is often ignored in primary care, the diagnosis of heart failure in most cases being based on symptoms and signs alone [11, 15, 16].

In addition, up to 50% of older heart failure patients have some degree of cognitive impairment [17], making history taking more difficult, more time-consuming and less reliable.

Decreased prevalence of key symptoms and signs

Exertional breathlessness, which is often regarded as an inevitable consequence of heart failure, occurs less frequently in older patients and, when present, tends to

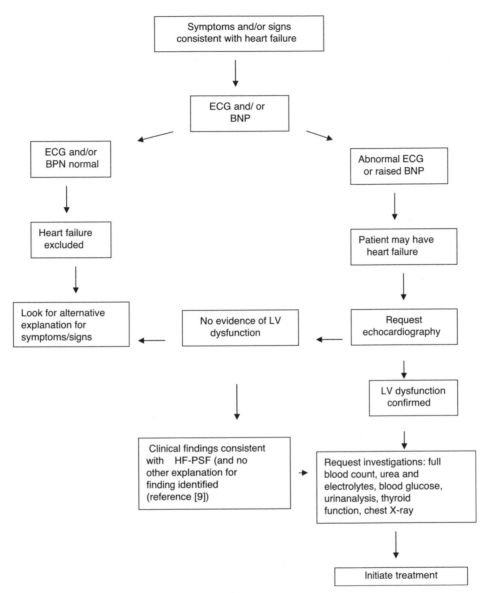

Figure 5.1 Algorithm: a process for the diagnosis of heart failure. (Based on data from Ref. [3].)

begin later in the course of the disease. There are several reasons for this. Some older people choose to exercise less than when they were younger or, having retired, do not substitute a leisure-time activity for the activity associated with their employment. In others, inactivity is imposed by comorbidities such as a stroke, intermittent claudication, arthritis or other musculoskeletal problems.

Orthopnoea and paroxysmal nocturnal dyspnoea are also less common, perhaps because their onset is delayed by age-related pulmonary vascular changes [13]. As with exertional breathlessness, if these symptoms do occur, it is often late in the course of the disease.

In addition, as noted above [5], classical clinical signs of a raised venous pressure, basal pulmonary crepitations, hepatomegaly and peripheral oedema are often absent, even in younger patients [5]. Yet, in older patients they are even less common, the sensitivity being less than 10% [11, 18]. This is partly a reflection of a failure to detect a sign which may actually be present, and partly because of the inclusion of patients who had only mild heart failure.

Atypical presenting symptoms

In older patients, the initial complaint may be a cough, lethargy, confusion, falls, dizziness or syncope, insomnia or anxiety, any of which may be attributed to an alternative cause or to 'old age' [13].

Attributing symptoms caused by heart failure to an alternative pathology, or vice versa

Some of the typical symptoms and signs of heart failure are easily confused with those of one or more of the comorbidities which characterize this age group (see Chapter 8 and Table 5.2):

- With respect to diagnosing heart failure in older patients, 'symptoms and signs consistent with the diagnosis' is more appropriate than 'specific symptoms and signs... of heart failure' as is required in published guidelines.

- Older patients who present with atypical or vague, ill-defined symptoms should undergo an ECG or BNP assay to exclude heart failure, unless an alternative explanation for their symptoms (other than 'old age') is clearly identified.

Failure to identify the correct aetiology

Three aetiologies in particular are easily overlooked in older patients [13, 18].

- Myocardial infarction often presents 'silently', as heart failure, without the characteristic chest pain.

- In aortic stenosis, the typically slow rising pulse character may be obscured by hypertension and the character of the murmur can be changed by the presence of atrial fibrillation, which is common; alternatively, it may be obscured by chronic obstructive pulmonary disease (COPD).

Table 5.2 Common symptoms and signs of heart failure which may be attributed to, or caused by, other conditions. (Heart failure commonly coexists with most of these conditions.)

Symptom	Alternative diagnoses
Exertional breathlessness	COPD[a], obesity, anaemia, deconditioning, pulmonary atelectasis
Peripheral oedema	Renal failure, arthritis, obesity, venous insufficiency
Fatigue/lethargy	Depression, anaemia, deconditioning
Reduced exercise tolerance	Arthritis, deconditioning, anaemia
Pulmonary crepitations	COPD, pulmonary atelectasis

[a]Chronic obstructive pulmonary disease.

- The murmur of acute-onset mitral regurgitation, which commonly presents as LV failure, may be insignificant. Also, as noted in Chapter 4, most patients with severe functional mitral regurgitation have no audible murmur.

In the light of these numerous difficulties it is not surprising that when heart failure is diagnosed in primary care the diagnosis is, more often than not, incorrect [19–21] and that, in genuine cases, it may often be overlooked or delayed.

The difficulties and delays in diagnosing heart failure in older patients have serious consequences (based on Ref. [13]):

- Hospitalization because of severe symptoms becomes more common.

- Standard medicines may be less effective because irreversible myocardial damage is more likely to occur.

- Secondary preventive measures may be less effective than if initiated sooner.

- Because of more extensive myocardial damage before treatment, morbidity and mortality are higher.

5.5 Diagnosis, patient management and clinical profile

Optimum treatment

Providing the optimum treatment for any condition depends on the accuracy of the diagnosis and, in the case of heart failure, on identifying the aetiology (see Chapter 4). Although a guideline-based optimized drug regimen is appropriate for the majority of patients, for others it needs to be modified to accommodate the treatment of coexisting conditions, or to address other heart failure-related problems. (It should be noted that the *Concise Oxford Dictionary* states that 'optimum' means 'best compromise': It is not synonymous with 'maxi-mum tolerated'.)

This need to compromise or modify treatment is particularly relevant for older patients:

- Older heart failure patients usually have several comorbidities (see Chapter 8), one or more of which may be the dominant clinical problem demanding priority treatment.

- Complications of heart failure develop more often in older patients; for example, there is a higher prevalence of atrial fibrillation, which requires additional or modified treatment.

- A decline in renal function is common, as a result of which treatment (e.g. with an ACE inhibitor) may have to be reduced or discontinued.

- Polypharmacy, because of comorbidities, often results in drug interactions or adverse side effects, and may preclude some medications.

Other factors must also be taken into account when deciding what constitutes 'optimum treatment': the aetiology (Chapter 4), a possible precipitant for heart failure, the severity of symptoms, or the results of baseline investigations.

Identification of a precipitant

Patients with heart failure usually seek attention because of breathlessness, fatigue or oedema that often results from slowly progressive LV dilatation and impairment. However, in some cases there is a specific precipitant (see Table 5.3 and Chapter 12), with myocardial ischaemia, atrial fibrillation and chest infection being the most common. Each precipitant must be addressed specifically, in conjunction with that of heart failure. In this respect, the use of the headings 'underlying', 'fundamental' and 'precipitating' to classify patients [22] (see Chapter 4) is a useful reminder of the need to seek a trigger for the patient's heart failure.

The severity of symptoms

Symptom severity, which is usually assessed by NYHA class (see Chapter 2), is relevant to the choice of treatment as well as to predicting the prognosis. For example, aldosterone receptor antagonists are recommended only for patients in NYHA class IV (see Chapter 6). In older, frail patients it can be difficult to assess the NYHA class as they are often quite inactive by choice, or they may have a noncardiac

Table 5.3 Common precipitants of heart failure or of cardiac deterioration.

Precipitant	Comments
Cardiac causes	
Myocardial infarction/ischaemia	May be clinically silent in older patients
Atrial fibrillation	Notably older hypertensive female patients
Other arrhythmias including heart block and sick sinus syndrome	
Medication-related causes	
Negative inotropes[a]	Avoid diltiazem/verapamil and anti-arrhythmic drugs other than amiodarone
NSAIDs, corticosteroids, lithium, tricyclic antidepressants	
Other medical causes	
Renal dysfunction	Increases with age, may be iatrogenic
Anaemia	Increases with age
Poorly controlled hypertension	Increases with age
Pulmonary embolism	
COPD $\pm$ chest infection	
Patient-related causes	
Noncompliance (note particular problems in the cognitively impaired)	
Alcohol abuse	

[a]Beta-blockers, although negatively inotropic, are safe if prescribed according to published guidelines (see Chapter 6).

comorbidity such as a musculoskeletal problem. In these patients it may be easier and more useful to assess functional status based on a description of their normal daily activities, using an 'activities of daily living' scale [23] rather than on the basis of NYHA class.

Baseline investigations

In addition to echocardiography, ECG and chest X-ray, a number of other baseline investigations should be routinely undertaken to check renal function prior to treatment with an ACE inhibitor, to identify comorbidities, and to screen for any side effects of medications (see Chapter 6 and Table 5.4).

With few exceptions, older patients have a complex clinical profile. Hence, as an aid to providing the optimum appropriate treatment, each relevant factor discussed should be identified and included as part of a patient's diagnostic profile.

Table 5.4 Routine baseline investigations.

Investigation	Purpose/function	Abnormality identified
ECG	Baseline, identify aetiology, pathology	Myocardial infarction, LV hypertrophy, arrhythmias
Chest X-ray	Baseline, diagnosis	Cardiomegaly, primary lung pathology
Full blood count	Baseline	Anaemia
Urea/electrolytes creatinine	Baseline, monitoring	Pre-existing renal disease/ dysfunction
Urinalysis	Baseline, diagnosis	Proteinuria (renal disease), diabetes
Thyroid function tests	Identify cause	Hyper/hypothyroidism as a cause of heart failure.
	Monitoring	Monitoring of amiodarone treatment
Lipid profile	Diagnosis	Hyperlipidaemia
Hepatic enzymes	Baseline, monitoring	For example, for drug toxicity (e.g. statins)

References

1. Swedberg, K., Cleland, J., Dargie, H. *et al.* (2005) Guidelines for the diagnosis and treatment of chronic heart failure: full text (update 2005). The Task Force for the diagnosis and treatment of CHF of the European Society of Cardiology. *European Heart Journal*, **26**, 1115–1140.

2. American College of Cardiology/American Heart Association (2005) Guideline update for the diagnosis and management of chronic heart failure in the adult. *Circulation*, **112**, 154–235.

3. Scottish Intercollegiate Guidelines Network (SIGN) (2007) *Management of chronic heart failure. A national clinical guideline*. Royal College of Physicians, Edinburgh. Available at www.sign.ac.uk.

4. Petrie, M.C. and McMurray, J.J.V. (2003) It cannot be cardiac failure because the heart is not enlarged on the chest X-ray. *The European Journal of Heart Failure*, **5**, 117–119.

5. Stevenson, L.W. and Perloff, J.K. (1989) The limited reliability of physical signs for estimating hemodynamics in chronic heart failure. *Journal of the American Medical Association*, **261** (6), 884–888.

6. Androne, A.S., Katz, S.D., Lund, L. *et al.* (2003) Hemodilution is common in patients with advanced heart failure. *Circulation*, **107**, 226–229.

7. McMurray, J., Komadja, M., Anker, S. and Gardner, R. (2006) Heart Failure: Epidemiology, Pathophysiology and Diagnosis, in *The European Society of Cardiology Textbook of*

Cardiovascular Medicine (eds J.A. Cramm, T.F. Luscher and P.W. Serryus), Blackwell Publishing, pp. 685–720.

8. Assoumull, R.G., Pennell, D.J. and Prasad, S.K. (2007) Cardiovascular magnetic resonance in the evaluation of heart failure. *Heart*, **93**, 985–992.

9. Vasan, R.S., Benjamin, E.J. and Levy, D. (1996) Congestive heart failure with normal left ventricular systolic function: Clinical approaches to the diagnosis and treatment of diastolic heart failure. *Archives of Internal Medicine*, **156** (2), 146–157.

10. Maisel, A.S., McCord, J., Nowak, R.M. *et al.* (2003) Bedside B type naturetic peptide in the emergency diagnosis of heart failure with reduced or preserved ejection fraction. *Journal of the American College of Cardiology*, **41**, 1252–1259.

11. Fonseca, C., Morais, H., Mota, T. *et al.* (2004) The diagnosis of heart failure in primary care: value of symptoms and signs. *European Journal of Heart Failure*, **6**, 795–800.

12. Tresch, D.D. (1997) The clinical diagnosis of heart failure in older patients. *Journal of the American Geriatric Society*, **45**, 1128–1133.

13. Tresch, DD. (1987) Atypical presentation of cardiovascular disorders in the elderly. *Geriatrics*, **42**, 31–46.

14. Rich, M.W. (2006) Heart failure in older people. *Medical Clinics of North America*, **90**, 863–885.

15. Hobbs, F.D.R., Jones, M.I., Allan, T.F. *et al.* (2000) European survey of primary care physicians perceptions on heart failure diagnosis and management (Euro-HF). *European Heart Journal*, **21**, 1877–1887.

16. Owen, A. and Cox, S. (2001) Diagnosis of heart failure in elderly patients in primary care. *European Journal of Heart Failure*, **3**, 79–81.

17. Zuccala, G., Cattel, C., Manes-Gravina, E. *et al.* (1997) Left ventricular dysfunction: A clue to cognitive impairment in older patients with heart failure. *Journal of Neurological and Neurosurgical Psychiatry*, **63**, 509–512.

18. Tresch, D.D. (1997) Atypical presentation of heart failure in older patients. *Journal of the American Geriatric Association*, **45** (9), 1128–1133.

19. Cowie, M.R., Struthers, A.D., Wood, D.A. *et al.* (1997) Value of naturetic peptides in assessment of patients with possible new heart failure in primary care. *The Lancet*, **350** (9088), 1349–1353.

20. Remes, J., Meittenen, H., Reunanen, A. *et al.* (1991) Validity of clinical diagnosis of heart failure in primary health care. *European Heart Journal*, **12**, 315–321.

21. Sparrow, N., Adlam, D., Cowley, A.S. *et al.* (2003) The diagnosis of heart failure in general practice: implications for the UK National Service Framework. *European Journal of Heart Failure*, **5**, 349–354.

22. Givertz, M.M., Colucci, W.S. and Braunwald, E. (2001) Clinical aspects of heart failure, in *Heart Disease, A. Textbook of Cardiovascular Medicine*, 6th edn (eds E. Braunwald, D.P. Zipes and P. Libby), W.B. Saunders Company, Ch. 17.

23. Lawton, M.P. and Brody, E.M. (1969) Assessment of older people: Self maintaining and instrumental activities of daily living. *Gerontologist*, **9**, 179–186.

6

Pharmacological treatment

Miles D. Witham

Section of Ageing and Health, Ninewells Hospital, Dundee

Key messages

- ACE inhibitors and beta-blockers are first-line therapies for all patients with LV systolic dysfunction, regardless of age and symptoms.

- The side effects of ACE inhibitors and beta-blockers are broadly similar, irrespective of patient age.

- Spironolactone and digoxin can be prescribed for patients with severe persistent symptoms, but carry high a risk of side effects in older people.

- Evidence for treating heart failure with preserved systolic function is weaker, but angiotensin receptor blockers, ACE inhibitors and some beta-blockers may improve symptoms and reduce hospitalization.

6.1   Introduction

Despite the large amount of high-quality trial evidence that now underpins prescribing for heart failure, there is ample evidence that many older people do not receive evidence-based drug therapy [1–3]. The reasons underlying this are considerably more complex than some commentators have suggested, however. In order to examine the issue of prescribing for older heart failure patients, a brief review of important factors bearing on prescribing is therefore in order.

A Practical Guide to Heart Failure in Older People, Edited by C Ward and M D Witham
© 2009 John Wiley & Sons, Ltd

What are the aims of therapy in older people?

Most clinicians caring for older people with heart failure would suggest that postponing death, reducing hospitalization, improving symptoms and exercise capacity, and improving quality of life are all important goals in caring for older heart failure patients. Those with an eye on the practice or hospital budget would add that containing the spiralling costs of caring for people with heart failure is another important goal.

There is, however, surprisingly little information regarding what older people themselves want from heart failure treatment [4–7]. The results of studies that do exist have suggested that, whilst some patients do indeed rate the prolongation of life very highly, a substantial minority rate symptom control as more important – even at the expense of prolonging life. Clearly, the wishes of each patient need to be ascertained on an individual basis.

Side effects versus benefits

The other half of the equation is the risk of side effects. Older people are more prone to side effects from any medication – the result of impaired organ function, reduced homeostatic reserve, comorbid disease and polypharmacy. The risk of a drug interaction causing a side effect rises exponentially with the number of medications taken, reaching 80% once 15 or more medications are taken – a not unusual situation in older people with many comorbidities.

Concordance

Several other barriers potentially exist to prevent older people from taking prescribed medications. Can they physically collect the medications? Does cognitive impairment make it difficult to remember when to take medications? Does the patient agree with the rationale for taking the medication – and does the patient wish to tolerate the side effects for the perceived level of benefit?

Problems with the evidence base

The other major factor to be considered in any discussion of drug intervention for older people is the applicability of the evidence base [8, 9]. Despite the majority of heart failure sufferers being aged 75 and over, the mean age of patients recruited into trials of heart failure treatment is usually much younger – typically between 50 and 70. Patients in trials often have little comorbid disease and are physically and cognitively more robust than typical patients; indeed, patients are often actively excluded if they have multiple comorbidities. Furthermore, many trials of heart failure focus on death and hospitalization as outcomes. Whilst these outcomes are important to some patients, symptoms and quality of life are at least as important for others.

The consequences of this skewed evidence base are manifold. First, there is uncertainty as to whether the degree of benefit seen in younger patients can be extrapolated to older patients. Second, the balance between risks and benefits in older people is unknown. A typical example would be whether the reduction in morbidity from heart failure from cardiovascularly active medication is negated by increased numbers of falls in frail older patients.

Third, the evidence of improvement in so-called 'soft' outcomes (exercise capacity, symptoms and quality of life) is often much less robust than for death and hospitalization. For those patients who place most value on these outcomes, the evidence needed to guide choice of therapy is therefore less strong.

6.2   ACE inhibitors

Angiotensin-converting enzyme inhibitors (ACEi) were one of the first classes of drug to demonstrate improvement in outcomes in patients with heart failure. The results of several large trials have demonstrated unequivocally that ACEi reduce mortality and hospitalization, as well as improving symptoms, in younger heart failure patients [10, 11]; these benefits appear to be independent of age [12].

Evidence in very old heart failure patients is lacking; the mean age of patients in large trials of ACEi was less than 65 years, and the prescribing of ACEi to older heart failure patients has for many years lagged behind rates for younger patients [13]. Concerns regarding falls, postural hypotension and even cognitive impairment were manifest, along with concern about exacerbating chronic kidney disease, which is highly prevalent among older patients.

Having said this, there is evidence that ACEi do improve exercise capacity in typical older heart failure patients [14], and the incidence of postural hypotension and dizziness is much less of a problem with long-acting ACEi than with captopril. Even traditional contraindications to ACEi may have been overstated; heart failure patients inadvertently started on ACEi with contraindications including aortic stenosis live longer than those not on ACEi [15], and ACEi may in fact improve exercise tolerance in severe aortic stenosis [16]. Today, ACEi have a central role in retarding the progression of chronic kidney disease and can improve exercise capacity even in older patients without heart failure [17].

Who should receive ACEi?

- All patients with LV systolic dysfunction, regardless of symptom level.

- All patients with other vascular disease (previous myocardial infarction, stroke or angina).

Which ACEi to use?

A long-acting ACE inhibitor is preferred, as there is less chance of post-dose hypotension, and the dose can be taken once per day, aiding adherence to therapy. Although debate continues as to the relative efficacy of different ACEi, persuasive evidence that anything other than a class effect is operating is lacking.

How should ACEi be started?

Nowadays, patients rarely need to attend hospital for ACEi treatment to be initiated. Before starting, care should be taken that the patient is not clinically dehydrated; a small reduction in diuretic therapy for a few days may be required. Baseline renal function and electrolytes should be checked.

A safe strategy is to start with the lowest dose available, and to increase this stepwise every two weeks, checking the blood pressure, renal function and electrolytes before each dose titration. The aim is to reach the highest recommended dose; the ATLAS trial [18] suggested that high doses of ACEi reduced hospitalization (but not mortality) more than low doses. Many older patients will not tolerate the highest recommended dose however, and if symptoms such as dizziness occur then the dosage should be returned to the previous titration step.

Contraindications to the use of ACEi are listed in Table 6.1. It is usual for the creatinine level to rise by up to 30% on starting ACEi treatment. However, if the creatinine increases by 50% or more [19], or rises to over $300\,\mu mol\,l^{-1}$, the ACEi should be stopped for a week, renal function rechecked, and the process of dose titration restarted at a lower dose. The possibility of renal artery stenosis should be considered if the creatinine rises dramatically on starting treatment. The potassium may also rise; an increase up to $5.9\,mmol\,l^{-1}$ is acceptable, but above this the ACE inhibitor should again be stopped for a week and reintroduced at a lower dose.

If a cough occurs on starting with an ACE inhibitor, it should be discontinued and an angiotensin receptor blocker substituted (see below). A careful clinical history is required for the patient however, as the cough may be due to existing lung disease (e.g. COPD), to intercurrent illness, or to pulmonary congestion – the result of heart failure.

Table 6.1 Contraindications to ACE inhibitors.

Previous angioedema with ACE inhibitors
Systolic BP <90 mmHg
Cough with ACE inhibitors
Severe aortic stenosis
Serum creatinine $>200\,\mu mol\,l^{-1}$
Serum potassium $>5.0\,mmol\,l^{-1}$

Many patients with severe heart failure have a low blood pressure, and it is difficult to give absolute cut-offs below which ACEi should be discontinued, or not started. A pragmatic approach is required – if the patient feels unwell, is tired or dizzy and has a very low blood pressure, then consider stopping the ACEi.

6.3 Beta-blockers

Beta-blocker therapy illustrates many of the aforementioned concerns about the applicability of the evidence base to older people. In younger people, excellent trial evidence suggests that beta-blockers reduce symptoms, reduce hospitalization and reduce mortality from heart failure. Until recently, such evidence was severely lacking in older people, but subgroup analyses of age groups in the CIBIS II and MERIT-HF trials suggests that benefit is still seen in those aged between 70 and 80 years.

In the recent SENIORS study [20], older people with heart failure were specifically enrolled, including patients with both preserved and impaired LV systolic function. Although the primary endpoint of reduced death and hospitalization was not reached, there was a statistically significant reduction in hospitalization. But - two words of caution are needed. The benefit in those patients with preserved LV function was less apparent, as was the benefit in the subgroup aged 75 and over. There is still no good evidence that very old heart failure patients obtain improved exercise capacity or quality of life from starting beta-blockers.

Many prescribers have been reluctant to give older people beta-blockers. Some of this reluctance perhaps stems from the fact that, until the mid-1990s, beta-blockers were felt to be contraindicated in heart failure (and were one of the stated reasons for failing medical students in finals exams at the author's medical school!). Alongside this requirement for a cultural shift in prescribing behaviour, prescribers had concerns regarding heart block, falls, fatigue and confusion in older people – concerns that the large randomized trials did nothing to allay. Studies of beta-blocker use in older people in practice have shown that tolerability is reasonable; approximately 70% of patients can tolerate a beta-blocker, albeit at a somewhat lower dose than younger heart failure patients [21–23].

Who should receive a beta-blocker?

Most guidelines now agree that all patients with LV systolic dysfunction should be receiving a beta-blocker. Contraindications to the use of beta-blockers are listed in Table 6.2.

It should be noted that many patients with COPD will be able to tolerate a beta-blocker – especially those without a large reversible component to their airways

Table 6.2   Contraindications to beta-blocker use.

Second- or third-degree heart block (unless pacemaker fitted)
Symptomatic hypotension (systolic BP <90 mmHg)
Asthma or COPD with a prominent reversible component
Decompensated heart failure (i.e. severe ankle oedema, pulmonary crackles)
Critical peripheral vascular disease

disease – and this group of patients was represented in the CIBIS II trial [24]. Disease severity on spirometry is not a good predictor of who will tolerate beta-blockade, and for many patients an empirical trial is necessary.

Which beta-blocker to use?

Bisoprolol, carvedilol and extended release metoprolol (not available in the UK) are licensed for use in heart failure and have good trial evidence supporting them. Nebivolol was used in the SENIORS trial and is an alternative. The choice of beta-blocker may be important; for example, the BEST study failed to find a survival benefit using bucindolol. There is no trial evidence to support use of atenolol or propranolol.

How should they be started?

Patients should not be fluid-overloaded, and thus adequate diuretic therapy is required. Starting beta-blockers in patients with fluid overload is likely to exacerbate the problem and may lead to acute decompensation of heart failure.

The chosen beta-blocker should be started at the lowest available dose and administered for at least two weeks before increasing the dose. Two typical dose titration schemes are shown in Table 6.3.

Table 6.3   Dose titration of beta-blockers.

	Bisoprolol	Carvediolol
Start	1.25 mg o.d.	3.125 mg b.d.
	2.5 mg o.d.	6.25 mg b.d.
	3.75 mg o.d.	12.5 mg b.d.
	5 mg o.d.	25 mg b.d.
	10 mg o.d.	(50 mg b.d. if mild symptoms and body weight >85 kg)

Titrate at 2–4-week intervals. If symptoms become problematic (fluid overload, dizziness, bradycardia <50 per min), step back a dose.

What should be done if side effects occur?

Transient tiredness and fatigue are common side effects of starting beta-blockade, and will often resolve, but the patient should be encouraged to persevere. Wheeze is more serious, and should prompt consideration of stopping beta-blockers, although care must be taken to determine whether the wheezing is due to bronchospasm or to pulmonary congestion.

If other side effects occur, the dose should be reduced back to the previous tolerated step on the titration scheme. If still not tolerated, then a different beta-blocker should be prescribed. A substantial minority of patients who are intolerant of one type of beta-blocker manage to tolerate a different type [21]. Low blood pressure alone is not necessarily a problem; it is more important to be guided by symptoms and by whether or not renal function is stable.

Is it better to give a beta-blocker or an ACE inhibitor first?

Although ACEi are usually commenced before beta-blockers, this probably reflects the order in which they were introduced into clinical practice for heart failure management. ACEi can usually be started earlier in decompensated heart failure, as they are well tolerated when fluid overload is present. There is evidence that introducing a beta-blocker first has beneficial effects on the LV ejection fraction and NYHA functional class [25], although the CIBIS III study showed no difference in mortality rates between those starting enalapril first and those starting bisoprolol first [26].

6.4 Spironolactone

The use of spironolactone has undergone a rebirth in recent years. No longer a humble potassium-sparing diuretic, its ability to block the many deleterious effects of aldosterone on the vascular system has provided it with a niche in heart failure management. The RALES trial [27] demonstrated a 30% reduction in death and hospitalization in patients with severe heart failure (LVEF <35% and NYHA class III and IV symptoms).

Unfortunately, the familiarity of many prescribers with spironolactone has led some to underestimate the potential for side effects and harm with this medication. Older people with heart failure (and the inevitable concomitant renal dysfunction) do not tolerate spironolactone well. In fact, some 25% have to discontinue the medication due to worsening renal function or hyperkalaemia, and 50% suffer from at least one side effect [28,29]. This incidence is much higher than that found in the carefully selected, younger subjects in the RALES trial [27]. The problem has been

Table 6.4 Contraindications to spironolactone use.

Serum potassium $>5.0\,\mathrm{mmol\,l^{-1}}$
Serum creatinine $>221\,\mathrm{\mu mol\,l^{-1}}$
Hypotension (systolic BP $<90\,\mathrm{mmHg}$)
Nonsevere symptoms
Mild LV systolic dysfunction

exacerbated by the use of spironolactone in patients with milder symptoms than were enrolled in the RALES trial; such patients may have less to gain, and thus the balance of benefit and risk tips away from using spironolactone. These factors may explain why no improvement in heart failure mortality was seen after introducing spironolactone in a large Canadian cohort [30].

Who should receive spironolactone?

Patients should have severe heart failure, with a LVEF <35% (i.e. moderate LV systolic dysfunction or worse) and severe symptoms (NYHA class III or IV), despite therapy with ACEi, beta-blockers and diuretics. Contraindications to the use of spironolactone are listed in Table 6.4. All patients in the RALES trial were taking ACEi; there is no evidence that aldosterone blockade in the absence of angiotensin blockade is effective.

How should spironolactone be used?

Spironolactone treatment should be started at a dose of 25 mg, once daily, although a few patients may require less (12.5 mg once daily). There is seldom any reason to increase the dose to 50 mg once daily, as this dose level is associated with a higher incidence of side effects. Occasionally, patients may require this higher dose to control persistent hypokalaemia, however.

The most important factor in using spironolactone safely is regular, frequent checks of potassium levels and renal function. This is particularly important whenever an intercurrent illness occurs; diarrhoeal illnesses are particularly notable for precipitating acute renal failure in patients taking spironolactone.

What should be done if side effects occur?

In most patients, side effects (especially renal dysfunction) will mean that the spironolactone treatment must be stopped. Although some patients (e.g. with intercurrent illness) can be restarted, most patients with renal dysfunction as a result of spironolactone will encounter the same problem a short time later [28].

Eplerenone is a new, selective aldosterone antagonist. As such, it avoids the side effect of gynaecomastia associated with spironolactone. However, patients taking eplerenone are still at risk of renal dysfunction and hyperkalaemia, and it is therefore not suitable as a replacement for most patients suffering side effects with spirono-lactone. Eplerenone is specifically indicated for patients who have a low LVEF after acute myocardial infarction [31], and does not currently have a licence for use in chronic heart failure *per se*.

6.5 Diuretics

Diuretics remain an important part of the therapeutic armamentarium for older heart failure patients, but should not be used at the expense of other heart failure medications. Whilst diuretics can dramatically improve symptoms due to fluid overload, they produce a high burden of side effects such as urinary frequency, incontinence, renal dysfunction, dizziness and falls.

Who should receive diuretics?

Diuretics should be given to any patient with fluid overload, especially with pulmo-nary congestion on chest X-ray, a raised jugular venous pressure (JVP) or ascites. Many patients receive diuretics for ankle swelling; this is justified if heart failure is the cause, but it is often ineffective and can lead to dehydration if the ankle swelling is due to other medications (e.g. calcium channel blockers) or venous insufficiency. There is now evidence from systematic reviews that diuretic therapy does indeed reduce the chances of death or hospitalization for heart failure [32]; such evidence has surprisingly been lacking until recently!

Patients without signs of fluid overload are unlikely to be helped symptomatically by starting or increasing diuretics; medications such as ACEi and beta-blockers are required to produce further symptomatic benefit in these patients.

Doses of diuretics

In a patient with normal renal and cardiac functions, an intravenous dose of 40 mg furosemide will produce a near-maximum diuresis; oral doses of 1 mg of the more bioavailable bumetanide and 20 mg of torasemide have similar effects. The loop diuretic dose required for maximum effect is, however, higher in patients with renal failure or heart failure, since in these settings decreased renal perfusion (and therefore decreased drug delivery to the kidney), diminished proximal secretion of diuretic (due to the retention of competing anions in renal failure) and enhanced activity of sodium-retaining forces (such as the renin-angiotensin-aldosterone system) combine to diminish the diuretic effect.

When considering appropriate diuretic dosage in older patients with heart failure, clinicians should therefore take into account the presence and degree of renal dysfunction. Single doses of 120 mg or more of intravenous furosemide, 5 mg or more of oral bumetanide, or 40 mg or more of torasemide may be necessary to achieve maximal diuresis. Salt and water homeostasis is however abnormal in a wide variety of ways in older, frailer patients, and despite the theoretical need to increase diuretic doses in patients with renal dysfunction it is clinically prudent to commence treatment with standard doses (40 mg furosemide) in this patient subgroup. Doses should be increased slowly; if twice-daily doses are used, an evening dose should be avoided if possible, as the resultant diuresis is likely to lead to disturbed sleep.

Resistant fluid overload

Fluid overload that is resistant to increasing doses of diuretics is often an indication for hospital admission (see Chapters 11 and 12) or at the least, specialist consultation. Intravenous diuretics are often needed, especially as gut oedema reduces oral absorption. Extended diuretic infusions may also be required, as may the combination of a loop agent with a thiazide such as metolazone to produce synergistic diuretic effects.

6.6   Digoxin

Despite over 200 years of documented use in heart failure, the role of digoxin remains controversial. Unlike most positive inotropic agents (which usually increase mortality), digoxin also limits heart rate, which may underpin some of its beneficial effects.

In patients with atrial fibrillation, digoxin still provides a useful option for controlling heart rate, especially in those with marked fluid overload in whom beta-blockade is not appropriate. The role of digoxin in heart failure patients in sinus rhythm is more difficult to establish. The DIG trial suggested that in severe, refractory heart failure, digoxin could improve symptoms and reduce hospitalization, but did not reduce mortality. Digoxin has therefore found a niche in most heart failure guidelines for improving symptoms in patients with severe, refractory heart failure despite optimum treatment with the standard evidence-based drug regimen, but who are in sinus rhythm.

Two important caveats are required in older people. First, older heart failure patients are at a considerably increased risk of digoxin toxicity, often as a result of drug interactions and impaired renal clearance. Second, digoxin has significant anticholinergic side effects which are often underappreciated. As such, it is a risk factor for both falls and delirium. These problems may explain why digoxin is one of the three drugs most likely to result in hospital admission due to an adverse drug effect [33], and may also explain the increased mortality rate seen in the subset of patients in the DIG trial with digoxin levels in the upper part of the normal range.

Who should receive digoxin?

- Patients who require rate control for atrial fibrillation and who cannot take a beta-blocker (either because of intolerance or because their heart failure is currently decompensated).

- Patients who are in sinus rhythm, but remain severely symptomatic despite receiving ACEi, beta-blockers or spironolactone.

6.7 Hydralazine and nitrates

The combination of nitrates and hydralazine was first shown to improve mortality rates and exercise tolerance when given to heart failure patients on digoxin and diuretics over 20 years ago, in the VHeFT study [34]. Nitrates act as nitric oxide donors and venodilators, reducing preload to the right side of the heart; hydralazine combats oxidative stress and also acts as an arteriodilator, reducing afterload and thus allowing an increased output by the left ventricle. The combination has fallen out of favour since the early 1990s, mostly because of the superiority of ACEi as shown in VHeFT 2 [35]. However, recent trial evidence [36] supports a role for the combination in patients of Afro-Caribbean extraction; here, the mortality rate was 40% lower in the group given fixed-dose nitrates plus hydralazine, hospitalizations were lower, and the quality of life was improved. This was despite most patients already taking beta-blockers or ACEi, and a significant proportion also taking spironolactone and digoxin. Once again, however, caution is needed in extrapolating these results to typical older patients, as the mean age of patients in this study was 57 years.

Thus, in older patients who cannot take ACEi or angiotensin receptor blockers (especially in those with significant renal impairment), nitrate and hydralazine represents a possible therapy for older patients with otherwise difficult-to-control symptoms, especially for patients of Afro-Caribbean extraction. Care is needed however, as the combination can lead to orthostatic hypotension, and hydralazine is associated with nausea and, less commonly, rashes. Treatment should be started at low doses: 25 mg long-acting nitrate plus 12.5 mg thrice daily hydralazine, aiming for a maximum of 50 mg nitrate plus 50 mg thrice daily hydralazine, as tolerated. Fixed-dose combinations are also available in some countries.

6.8 Adding angiotensin receptor blockers to ACE inhibitors

Patients receiving chronic ACE inhibitor therapy suffer from an escape phenomenon, whereby the body finds other ways to enhance angiotensin II production. Several studies have therefore examined whether adding an angiotensin receptor blocker (ARB) to an ACE inhibitor leads to more complete blockade, with ensuing clinical benefits.

Trials, including CHARM and ValHEFT [37, 38], have now shown that the addition of an ARB to ACE inhibition further reduces mortality and hospitalization in patients with heart failure and impaired systolic function. However, the patients were relatively young (mean age 64 years in CHARM), and significant increases in hypotension and renal impairment were seen in the treatment arm. It is not clear whether most older heart failure patients are able to tolerate the addition of an ARB in addition to ACE inhibition, but for relatively younger, fitter patients it can be considered as a therapeutic option.

6.9 Treating the underlying cardiovascular disease

It is important to remember that almost all patients with chronic heart failure will have coexistent coronary, cerebral and/or peripheral vascular disease. Attention should thus be paid to secondary prevention with aspirin and statins, not forgetting the use of warfarin for patients in atrial fibrillation, unless contraindicated.

6.10 Medications to avoid

NSAIDs

Non-steroidal anti-inflammatory drugs (NSAIDs) cause fluid retention, thus worsening heart failure, and antagonize the effect of diuretics. They increase hypertension and may also increase the risk of cardiovascular events [39, 40]. They also worsen renal function, especially in combination with ACEi. Finally, NSAIDs are often ineffective as analgesics, and carry a high risk of gastrointestinal ulceration in older people. There is a strong case for never using NSAIDs in older people, and especially in older people with heart failure.

Calcium channel blockers

Heart rate-limiting calcium channel blockers (e.g. verapamil, diltiazem) are nega-tively inotropic, and as such may worsen heart failure and should generally be avoided. If heart rate control is required, then beta-blockers or digoxin are better options. The more newly introduced dihydropyridine-type calcium channel blockers (e.g. amlodipine) appear neutral in terms of mortality in heart failure, but can worsen ankle oedema. It may be necessary to use them for refractory angina or hypertension, but beta-blockers and nitrates are better options for angina, and ACEi, spironolactone and diuretics are better options for hypertension in patients with heart failure.

Class I anti-arrhythmics

All class I anti-arrhythmics (e.g. flecainide) are strongly negatively inotropic, and should therefore be avoided, as they can worsen heart failure. They are also pro-arrhythmic agents – that is they lead to an increase in the incidence of ventricular tachycardia which may prove fatal [41]. Interestingly, quinine has weak class I activity, yet is commonly prescribed for cramp in older people. It is not known whether this drug worsens the symptoms of heart failure or increases mortality or hospitalization. Similarly, tricyclic antidepressants have class I activity. Selective serotonin reuptake inhibitor (SSRI) antidepressants are less cardiotoxic and are probably a better choice for treating depression in patients with heart failure.

Thiazolidinediones

Thiazolidinediones (glitazones) cause fluid retention and are associated with a higher rate of heart failure diagnoses in clinical trials. They should therefore be avoided in patients with known heart failure.

Corticosteroids

Whilst it may not always be possible to avoid the use of steroids in older people with inflammatory conditions, they increase the risk of cardiovascular events [42] and cause fluid retention. If they have to be used, the dose should be as low as is needed, and for as short a time as possible. Increased doses of diuretics should be anticipated and started early.

Lithium

Lithium concentrations can be increased to dangerous levels by worsening renal function; the sodium depletion caused by diuretics can also worsen toxicity. Lithium is therefore best avoided in patients with heart failure.

6.11 Prescribing for heart failure with preserved systolic function

All of the above discussion applies to heart failure with impaired systolic function. By comparison, there is very little evidence to guide prescribing in patients with preserved systolic function heart failure, who comprise approximately 50% of all older heart failure patients.

There is general consensus that hypertension should be well controlled, as uncontrolled hypertension leads to LV hypertrophy that is often the substrate for heart failure with preserved function. Atrial fibrillation should also be controlled, as a rapid ventricular rate does not allow time for adequate ventricular filling.

Beyond this, three therapies – candesartan, perindopril and nebivolol – are worthy of consideration. Candesartan was shown to reduce hospitalization (but not mortality) in patients with preserved LV function (mean age 67 years) [43]. The PEP-CHF trial [44] enrolled older patients with (mean age 76) with preserved systolic function heart failure and comorbid disease, and although it failed to show an improvement in mortality, significant improvements in exercise capacity, symptom class and hospitalizations were seen in the group given perindopril. The SENIORS trial [20] included a number of patients with preserved LV function; a subgroup analysis suggested similar outcomes in those patients with mild impairment/preserved function when compared to patients with moderate/severe LV impairment. Observational studies suggest that patients with preserved LV function heart failure have improved survival when taking ACE inhibitors and/or beta-blockers [45].

Diuretic therapy is often required in patients with heart failure and preserved LV function. Care is needed to avoid overdiuresis, however, as many patients require reasonable filling pressures to allow a poorly relaxing hypertrophied ventricle to fill, and overdiuresis can lead to a precipitous fall in blood pressure.

6.12 Prescribing for multiple comorbidities

Heart failure rarely presents alone in older people, and the challenge is often to prescribe appropriately whilst minimizing the total number of medications to which the patient is exposed. Fortunately, it is often possible to combine medications to treat multiple problems (Table 6.5).

Table 6.5 Medications to treat combinations of comorbidity.

Comorbid condition	Suggested treatments
Hypertension	ACE inhibitors, ARBs, diuretics, beta-blockers
Angina	Beta-blockers, nitrates
Atrial fibrillation	Beta-blockers, digoxin

6.13 Prescribing at the end of life

Although, inevitably, there comes a point where medication to prolong life becomes inappropriate, diuretics and ACEi may still have a role as they reduce breathlessness. Other medications may need to be withdrawn, however. For intractable breathlessness, morphine and other opiates can provide effective relief, not only by reducing the sensation of breathlessness, but by also acting as venodilators (see also Chapter 14).

References

1. Cleland, J.G., Cohen-Solal, A., Aguilar, J.C. *et al.* (2002) Management of heart failure in primary care (the IMPROVEMENT of Heart Failure Programme): an international survey. *Lancet*, **360**, 1631–1639.
2. Heckman, G.A., Misiaszek, B., Merali, F. *et al.* (2004) Management of heart failure in Canadian long-term care facilities. *The Canadian Journal of Cardiology*, **20**, 963–969.
3. Murphy, N.F., Simpson, C.R., McAlister, F.A. *et al.* (2004) National survey of the prevalence, incidence, primary care burden, and treatment of heart failure in Scotland. *Heart (British Cardiac Society)*, **90**, 1129–1136.
4. Stanek, E.J., Oates, M.B., McGhan, W.F. *et al.* (2000) Preferences for treatment outcomes in patients with heart failure: symptoms versus survival. *Journal of Cardiac Failure*, **6**, 225–232.
5. Fried, T.R., Bradley, E.H. and Towle, V.R. (2003) Valuing the outcomes of treatment: do patients and their caregivers agree? *Archives of Internal Medicine*, **163**, 2073–2078.
6. Haydar, Z.R., Lowe, A.J., Kahveci, K.L. *et al.* (2004) Differences in end-of-life preferences between congestive heart failure and dementia in a medical house calls program. *Journal of the American Geriatrics Society*, **52**, 736–740.
7. Formiga, F., Chivite, D., Ortega, C. *et al.* (2004) End-of-life preferences in elderly patients admitted for heart failure. *Quarterly Journal of Medicine: Monthly Journal of the Association of Physicians*, **97**, 803–808.
8. Masoudi, F.A., Havranek, E.P., Wolfe, P. *et al.* (2003) Most hospitalized older persons do not meet the enrollment criteria for clinical trials in heart failure. *American Heart Journal*, **146**, 250–257.
9. McMurray, J. (2000) Heart failure: we need more trials in typical patients. *European Heart Journal*, **21**, 699–700.
10. The CONSENSUS Trial Study Group (1987) Effects of enalapril on mortality in severe congestive heart failure. Results of the Cooperative North Scandinavian Enalapril Survival Study (CONSENSUS). *The New England Journal of Medicine*, **316**, 1429–1435.
11. The SOLVD Investigators (1991) Effect of enalapril on survival in patients with reduced left ventricular ejection fractions and congestive heart failure. *New England Journal of Medicine*, **325** (5), 293–302.
12. Garg, R. and Yusuf, S. (1995) Overview of randomized trials of angiotensin-converting enzyme inhibitors on mortality and morbidity in patients with heart failure. Collaborative

Group on ACE Inhibitor Trials. *The Journal of the American Medical Association*, **273**, 1450–1456.

13. de Groote, P., Isnard, R., Assyag, P. *et al.* (2007) Is the gap between guidelines and clinical practice in heart failure treatment being filled? Insights from the IMPACT RECO survey. *European Journal of Heart Failure*, **9**, 1205–1211.

14. Hutcheon, S.D., Gillespie, N.D., Crombie, I.K. *et al.* (2002) Perindopril improves six minute walking distance in older patients with left ventricular systolic dysfunction: a randomised double blind placebo controlled trial. *Heart (British Cardiac Society)*, **88**, 373–377.

15. Ahmed, A., Kiefe, C.I., Allman, R.M. *et al.* (2002) Survival benefits of angiotensin-converting enzyme inhibitors in older heart failure patients with perceived contra-indications. *Journal of the American Geriatrics Society*, **50**, 1659–1666.

16. Chockalingam, A., Venkatesan, S., Subramaniam, T. *et al.* (2004) Safety and efficacy of angiotensin-converting enzyme inhibitors in symptomatic severe aortic stenosis: Symptomatic Cardiac Obstruction-Pilot Study of Enalapril in Aortic Stenosis (SCOPE-AS). *American Heart Journal*, **147**, E19.

17. Sumukadas, D., Witham, M.D., Struthers, A.D. and McMurdo, M.E. (2007) Effect of perindopril on physical function in elderly people with functional impairment: a randomized controlled trial. *Canadian Medical Association Journal*, **177**, 867–874.

18. Packer, M., Poole-Wilson, P.A., Armstrong, P.W. *et al.* (1999) Comparative effects of low and high doses of the angiotensin-converting enzyme inhibitor, lisinopril, on morbidity and mortality in chronic heart failure. ATLAS Study Group. *Circulation*, **100**, 2312–2318.

19. McMurray, J., Cohen-Solal, A., Dietz, R. *et al.* (2001) Practical recommendations for the use of ACE inhibitors, beta-blockers and spironolactone in heart failure: putting guidelines into practice. *European Journal of Heart Failure*, **3**, 495–502.

20. Flather, M.D., Shibata, M.C., Coats, A.J. *et al.* (2005) Randomized trial to determine the effect of nebivolol on mortality and cardiovascular hospital admission in elderly patients with heart failure (SENIORS). *European Heart Journal*, **26**, 215–225.

21. Witham, M.D., Gillespie, N.D. and Struthers, A.D. (2004) Age is not a significant risk factor for failed trial of beta-blocker therapy in older patients with chronic heart failure. *Age and Ageing*, **33**, 467–472.

22. Krum, H., Hill, J., Fruhwald, F. *et al.* (2006) Tolerability of beta-blockers in elderly patients with chronic heart failure: the COLA II study. *European Journal of Heart Failure*, **8**, 302–307.

23. Baxter, A.J., Spensley, A., Hildreth, A. *et al.* (2002) Beta blockers in older persons with heart failure: tolerability and impact on quality of life. *Heart (British Cardiac Society)*, **88**, 611–614.

24. CIBIS-II (1999) The Cardiac Insufficiency Bisoprolol Study II (CIBIS-II): a randomised trial. *Lancet*, **353**, 9–13.

25. Sliwa, K., Norton, G.R., Kone, N. *et al.* (2004) Impact of initiating carvedilol before angiotensin-converting enzyme inhibitor therapy on cardiac function in newly diagnosed heart failure. *Journal of the American College of Cardiology*, **44**, 1825–1830.

26. Willenheimer, R., van Veldhuisen, D.J., Silke, B. *et al.* (2005) Effect on survival and hospitalization of initiating treatment for chronic heart failure with bisoprolol followed by enalapril, as compared with the opposite sequence: results of the randomized Cardiac Insufficiency Bisoprolol Study (CIBIS) III. *Circulation,* **112,** 2426–2435.

27. Pitt, B., Zannad, F., Remme, W.J. *et al.* (1999) The effect of spironolactone on morbidity and mortality in patients with severe heart failure. Randomized Aldactone Evaluation Study Investigators. *The New England Journal of Medicine,* **341,** 709–717.

28. Witham, M.D., Gillespie, N.D. and Struthers, A.D. (2004) Tolerability of spironolactone in patients with chronic heart failure – a cautionary message. *British Journal of Clinical Pharmacology,* **58,** 554–557.

29. Dinsdale, C., Wani, M., Steward, J., O'Mahony and M.S. (2005) Tolerability of spironolactone as adjunctive treatment for heart failure in patients over 75 years of age. *Age and Ageing,* **34,** 395–398.

30. Juurlink, D.N., Mamdani, M.M., Lee, D.S. *et al.* (2004) Rates of hyperkalemia after publication of the Randomized Aldactone Evaluation Study. *The New England Journal of Medicine,* **351,** 543–551.

31. Pitt, B., Remme, W., Zannad, F. *et al.* (2003) Eplerenone, a selective aldosterone blocker, in patients with left ventricular dysfunction after myocardial infarction. *The New England Journal of Medicine,* **348,** 1309–1321.

32. Faris, R., Flather, M.D., Purcell, H. *et al.* (2006) Diuretics for heart failure. *Cochrane Database of Systematic Reviews,* CD003838.

33. Budnitz, D.S., Shehab, N., Kegler, S.R. and Richards, C.L. (2007) Medication use leading to emergency department visits for adverse drug events in older adults. *Annals of Internal Medicine,* **147,** 755–765.

34. Cohn, J.N., Archibald, D.G., Ziesche, S. *et al.* (1986) Effect of vasodilator therapy on mortality in chronic congestive heart failure. Results of a Veterans Administration Cooperative Study. *The New England Journal of Medicine,* **314,** 1547–1552.

35. Cohn, J.N., Johnson, G., Ziesche, S. *et al.* (1991) A comparison of enalapril with hydralazine-isosorbide dinitrate in the treatment of chronic congestive heart failure. *The New England Journal of Medicine,* **325,** 303–310.

36. Taylor, A.L., Ziesche, S., Yancy, C. *et al.* (2004) Combination of isosorbide dinitrate and hydralazine in blacks with heart failure. *The New England Journal of Medicine,* **351,** 2049–2057.

37. McMurray, J.J., Ostergren, J., Swedberg, K. *et al.* (2003) Effects of candesartan in patients with chronic heart failure and reduced left-ventricular systolic function taking angiotensin-converting-enzyme inhibitors: the CHARM-Added trial. *Lancet,* **362,** 767–771.

38. Cohn, J.N. and Tognoni, G. (2001) A randomized trial of the angiotensin-receptor blocker valsartan in chronic heart failure. *The New England Journal of Medicine,* **345,** 1667–1675.

39. Hippisley-Cox, J. and Coupland, C. (2005) Risk of myocardial infarction in patients taking cyclo-oxygenase-2 inhibitors or conventional non-steroidal anti-inflammatory

drugs: population based nested case-control analysis. *British Medical Journal (Clinical Research Ed.)*, **330**, 1366.

40. MacDonald, T.M. and Wei, L. (2006) Is there an interaction between the cardiovascular protective effects of low-dose aspirin and ibuprofen? *Basic and Clinical Pharmacology and Toxicology*, **98**, 275–280.

41. The Cardiac Arrhythmia Suppression Trial (CAST) Investigators. (1989) Preliminary report: effect of encainide and flecainide on mortality in a randomized trial of arrhythmia suppression after myocardial infarction. *The New England Journal of Medicine*, **321**, 406–412.

42. Wei, L., MacDonald, T.M. and Walker, B.R. (2004) Taking glucocorticoids by prescription is associated with subsequent cardiovascular disease. *Annals of Internal Medicine*, **141**, 764–770.

43. Yusuf, S., Pfeffer, M.A., Swedberg, K. *et al.* (2003) Effects of candesartan in patients with chronic heart failure and preserved left-ventricular ejection fraction: the CHARM-Preserved Trial. *Lancet*, **362**, 777–781.

44. Cleland, J.G., Tendera, M., Adamus, J. *et al.* (2006) The perindopril in elderly people with chronic heart failure (PEP-CHF) study. *European Heart Journal*, **27**, 2338–2345.

45. Shah, R., Wang, Y. and Foody, J.M. (2008) Effect of statins, angiotensin-converting enzyme inhibitors, and beta blockers on survival in patients > or = 65 years of age with heart failure and preserved left ventricular systolic function. *The American Journal of Cardiology*, **101**, 217–222.

7

Non-pharmacological management

Sinéad P. McKee[1] and Miles D. Witham[2]

[1] *Stirling Royal Infirmary, Livilands Gate, Stirling*
[2] *Section of Ageing and Health, Ninewells Hospital, Dundee*

Key messages

- Regular physical activity should be encouraged; structured exercise programmes improve outcomes for the 'younger' old heart failure patient.

- Smokers with heart failure should be urged to quit smoking.

- Excessive alcohol consumption should be avoided; heavy drinkers should abstain. Excessive salt and fluid consumption should be discouraged.

Although great advances have been made over the past 20 years in the management of heart failure, the majority of these have focussed on new pharmacological (and more recently device) therapies. Nevertheless, drugs bring with them side effects, and non-pharmacological interventions have an important part to play in managing heart failure in older people. Once again, the evidence base for such interventions is less firm than for drug interventions, and is less firm for older people than for younger people.

7.1 Exercise training

Twenty years ago, the conventional wisdom was that patients with heart failure should avoid undue exertion, and that the presence of chronic heart failure was a

---

A Practical Guide to Heart Failure in Older People, Edited by C Ward and M D Witham
© 2009 John Wiley & Sons, Ltd

contraindication to taking part in exercise training. Small studies of patients undertaking maximal exertion after large anterior myocardial infarction suggested that such strenuous exercise worsened overall myocardial function by exacerbating the difference in movement between the healthy and the damaged left ventricular (LV) walls.

Over the past two decades, however, the results of extensive research investigations have overturned this paradigm such that we now know that exercise training is safe, improves symptoms, quality of life [1] and, according to at least one meta-analysis, reduces death and hospitalization of patients with LV systolic dysfunction by approximately 25% [2].

Whilst this is excellent news for heart failure patients, a number of obstacles remain to be overcome in translating these research findings into benefits for older heart failure patients. Almost all of the studies on exercise training in heart failure have been conducted in relatively young patients with little comorbid disease, and often involves relatively intensive (three to five times per week) exercise using high-tech equipment such as bicycle ergometers and treadmills [1]. Such exercise programmes are clearly not suitable for the average older heart failure patient who comes equipped with arthritis, a catheter bag, two walking sticks and lives in a small flat!

Furthermore, almost all research performed to date has been conducted on patients with LV systolic dysfunction. It is therefore not clear whether the research findings extrapolate to the 50% of older heart failure patients with preserved LV function.

Having outlined these limitations, what practical advice can be given with regards to exercise training? There is no reason for heart failure patients to curtail their physical activity, as long as they are guided by their symptoms. Regular, preferably daily bouts of activity – especially walking – are likely to be beneficial, as long as dizziness or breathlessness do not become incapacitating. Patients should be told that a degree of breathlessness and fatigue on exertion is expected, and that is not a reason to avoid exertion. On the other hand, patients should avoid exertion to the point of exhaustion. If the patient cannot talk, they are exerting themselves too much and should slow down or stop for a little while [3].

7.2   Types of exercise programme

Exercise can include aerobic and/or resistance exercise. The target intensity for resistance exercise is no more than 80% of maximum; aerobic intensities of 50–80% of maximum (corresponding roughly to breathless but still able to talk) have been found to be safe and effective in younger patients [1]. For younger patients with relatively few comorbid diseases, suitable exercise programmes are now run in many cardiac rehabilitation centres; such programmes are also effective for the younger old [4]. It is not yet clear what format of exercise programmes are practical and effective for very old, frail patients; it is, however, clear that very gentle seated exercise is not effective at improving exercise capacity or quality of life [5]. Programmes involving stretching without significant aerobic or resistance work are unlikely to have any useful effect.

There are theoretical reasons for avoiding swimming in patients with significant heart failure symptoms; immersion of the thorax can have adverse effects on afterload and preload by increasing intrathoracic pressure, thus reducing cardiac output still further. Walking, golf, bowls, cycling and other everyday activities are safe, however.

Supervision

Early exercise programmes for patients with heart failure were heavily supervised, with continuous ECG recording and regular pulse and BP checks. As evidence has accumulated of the safety of such programmes, it has become clear that such precautions are not necessary – and may indeed even discourage patients from exercising, as they promote the perception that it is a hazardous activity. Almost all exercise programmes involve at least an initial supervised period, led by an experienced cardiac rehabilitation nurse or physiotherapist; this is desirable to ensure safety by instilling correct technique, encourage goal setting and to help overcome physical and psychosocial barriers to exercise [6, 7]. It is clear that the benefits of exercise are maintained only as long as exercise is maintained [8]; thus, programmes which allow participants to continue doing exercises unsupervised at home are essential for long-term efficacy.

Contraindications

Patients with acutely decompensated heart failure, severe aortic stenosis or intercurrent infection should not take part in exercise training (see Table 7.1). Any other contraindications are relative; if an exercise programme for older people is to be

Table 7.1 Contraindications to exercise training.

Unstable angina or myocardial infarction <6 weeks
Decompensated HF (pulmonary oedema or NYHA class IV symptoms)
Uncontrolled atrial fibrillation (ventricular rate >100 per min at rest)
Intercurrent infection
Severe aortic stenosis
History of sustained ventricular tachycardia or ventricular fibrillation outside the context of acute myocardial infarction

successful, it should be adaptable so that it is relevant to those who have comorbid disease, or difficulties with access and transport that often arise in older people. If exercise brings on chest pain suggestive of angina, then anti-anginal medications or further investigation are required.

Cognitive impairment is common in older heart failure patients, and although it is not an absolute contraindication to exercise training, it may make engagement with training more difficult, especially when training is to be continued in an unsupervised environment, for example the home.

Alternatives to exercise training are being examined for those who are unable to exercise (e.g. electrical muscle stimulation may have similar effects to exercise [9]). Evidence in very old heart failure patients is lacking, but such approaches may in future form an alternative to exercise for those who are chairbound or otherwise unable to exercise. Similarly, respiratory muscle training devices have met with success in some studies [10, 11], although the evidence is not as strong as for a whole-body approach to exercise training.

7.3   Smoking

Smoking cessation should be encouraged for two reasons. First, because in patients who smoke the heart rate and blood pressure are raised, contributing to increased myocardial oxygen consumption and increasing the chances of further myocardial ischaemic events that can worsen heart failure. Second, and more pertinently for many heart failure patients with compromised exercise capacity, smoking impairs the exercise capacity by reducing oxygen transport. Worsening lung function, peripheral vascular disease, intercurrent chest infections and the effects of carbon monoxide all conspire to make tiredness and breathlessness worse. Patients will see an improvement in exercise capacity within four weeks of giving up. Patients with heart failure who continue to smoke have higher rates of hospitalization and death than ex-smokers with heart failure [12]. The recently published EuroHeart Failure Survey II [13] showed that 15% of all patients admitted with acutely decompensated heart failure (mean age 70) were currently smoking.

What methods can be used to help?

Myocardial ischaemia – the most common aetiology of heart failure in older people – is a relative contraindication to nicotine replacement. However, nicotine replacement can be used in patients with stable coronary artery disease and no history of ventricular arrhythmia. Although a small risk of precipitating further ischaemic events is present, this may well be outweighed by the risks of continuing to smoke.

Although bupropion is not contraindicated in heart failure, there are several obstacles to its use in many older people, including renal impairment, the use of other medications that lower the seizure threshold (e.g. other antidepressants) and other interacting medications (e.g. L-dopa).

Counselling and education remain the cornerstone of smoking cessation in older heart failure patients, as in smokers of all ages. The presence of severe symptoms, and the significant improvements to be gained in the short term by stopping smoking, can be used as additional motivators for some heart failure patients. The specialist nurse and general practitioner can facilitate this process by reiterating the risks of continued smoking and assessing where the patient is in the behavioural cycle of change. If they are in the 'contemplation' or 'preparation' phase, then smoking cessation services should be involved. Positive reinforcement can be provided by all members of the multidisciplinary team.

7.4   Diet

There is surprisingly little information available to guide advice on diet for patients with heart failure. Randomized controlled trials are almost nonexistent, even for commonly used interventions such as sodium restriction.

Salt and fluid

Given that sodium and water retention are important factors in the decompensation of heart failure, the restriction of salt and fluid intake would be expected to reduce fluid retention. Whilst there is some evidence to support this [14], an overzealous approach is likely to fail in older people for the following reasons:

- Many older people have a heavily ingrained habit of adding salt to food, and compliance with advice to reduce salt intake is poor. Aiming for a daily salt intake of less than 6 g is reasonable, however, as recommended in the population-wide guidelines for the UK.

- Older people are prone to dehydration, especially if also taking diuretics. This can quickly lead to renal impairment, with the consequent build up of other drugs and eventually to hospital admission. It is wise to curtail excessive fluid intake (to less than 1.5 l per day) if fluid retention is problematic, but restriction beyond this is rarely successful.

Practical ways to reduce salt intake, such as not adding it at the table or while cooking, should be encouraged. Foods which are high in salt, such as peanuts, crisps, processed foods and ready-made convenience meals, should be avoided. It may be difficult for some older people to prepare their own meals and they may rely on convenience foods or meals prepared by others. Encouraging them to reduce snacks with a high salt content will be beneficial, and involving carers and relatives in counselling about food preparation and intake is therefore vital.

Daily weight monitoring can help patients detect early signs of fluid retention and clinical deterioration. Patients should be encouraged to record their weight at the same time each morning, using the same scales. This should be carried out prior to dressing or consuming any food, and after voiding. Of course, this is easier said than done for many older people, and patients who have limited mobility, visual problems or cognitive impairment will require help with monitoring their weight.

It is important for action to be taken on significant changes – there is little point recording it otherwise. An unexpected weight gain or loss of 2 kg or more over two days should be reported to the specialist nurse or general practitioner. Weight gain usually suggests fluid retention, while weight loss may be suggestive of dehydration; either way, an adjustment of diuretics and/or fluid intake will be required. Although some patients can be taught to adjust their own diuretics depending on changes in their weight, this approach should be used very carefully in older patients, where complicated drug regimes and polypharmacy can affect drug compliance.

Potassium

Many patients with heart failure have a degree of renal impairment, and are also taking medications (ACE inhibitors and spironolactone) that cause potassium retention. An excessive potassium intake (e.g. in salt substitutes) is therefore potentially dangerous, and should in general be avoided.

A few patients, especially those on large doses of loop diuretics and thiazides, may have low potassium levels; these patients may benefit from extra potassium in their diet.

Calorie intake

Whilst many older people with heart failure are obese [15], a few have cardiac cachexia, a condition that carries a particularly poor prognosis. Some patients – notably those with preserved systolic function who are overweight – seem to have a better prognosis than heart failure patients of normal weight [16]. This is despite obesity being a risk factor for coronary heart disease, and also being an important independent cause of reduced exercise capacity and breathlessness.

No randomized controlled trials have been conducted to guide interventions in this area. Although weight loss would be expected to improve exercise capacity and breathlessness, it seems that it could also worsen prognosis. Given these doubts, it is probably sensible to ensure that overweight heart failure patients do not gain further weight, reduce their saturated fat intake, and eat plenty of fruit and vegetables. Vigorous dieting should probably be avoided, pending further data in this area. Similarly, patients with unplanned weight loss should be referred to dietetic services for nutritional support, and may require further investigations to exclude any underlying malignancy.

Micronutrients and vitamins

A number of micronutrient and vitamin deficiencies have been associated with heart failure, including thiamine [17] and vitamin D [18]. Other micronutrients, for example coenzyme Q_{10}, are claimed to have beneficial effects in heart failure. There are mechanistic reasons for considering that the correction of some of these deficiencies may improve cardiac function and skeletal muscle function, and therefore symptoms and exercise capacity. One study of a multivitamin supplementation in older heart failure patients [19] did indeed show an improvement in LV function and quality of life, but not in exercise capacity. A small effect on systolic function was shown in a meta-analysis of trials of coenzyme Q_{10} [20], though whether this translates into a clinically meaningful effect is unclear. At present, research is ongoing in this area, and so it is difficult to provide any clear advice. However, a healthy, balanced diet, with plenty of fresh fruit and vegetables, is (as usual!) sound general advice.

7.5 Alcohol

Some older patients with heart failure drink alcohol to excess, and whilst this is rarely the only aetiology, it is often a contributory factor. Not only is alcohol itself a myocardial depressant, but the poor diet on which most heavy drinkers subsist may also lead to vitamin deficiencies, particularly of vitamin B_1, that are also associated with heart failure.

Small quantities of alcohol (1–2 units per day) are unlikely to be harmful for most heart failure patients, but for heavy drinkers abstinence should be advised. In some cases, this may lead to an improvement in cardiac function over time. It is also important for patients to include their alcohol volume in their daily fluid allowance. Moreover, alcohol contains additional calories that should be taken into consideration by those patients who need to lose weight.

For patients who have alcohol-induced cardiomyopathy, complete abstinence from alcohol is recommended. For this, specific counselling from an Alcohol Liaison Service, if available, may be required. Patients who take warfarin and who have a variable alcohol intake may have unstable anticoagulant control. It is safer to avoid alcohol in this situation.

7.6   Vaccinations

Pneumococcal and influenza infections can precipitate decompensation of heart failure symptoms, particularly in older patients. A large US cohort study [21] demonstrated a 37% reduction in hospital admissions for heart failure in community-dwelling older patients following an annual influenza vaccination. Patients should therefore be encouraged to receive the influenza vaccination and a one-off pneumococcal vaccination. The utilization of district nursing services may be required for those patients who are housebound.

7.7   Psychological interventions

Depression is very common in older people with any comorbid disease, and is especially common in patients with heart failure. Some studies have suggested that depression is an independent predictor of hospitalization and death from heart failure. There is, therefore, good reason to look for depression in patients with heart failure. Having identified depression however, there is no evidence to guide treatment, as no trials of antidepressants or psychological interventions have been conducted specifically in heart failure patients [22], and evidence from patients without heart failure must therefore be extrapolated. It is possible that both cognitive-behavioural therapy and antidepressants (but not tricyclic antidepressants) have their place here, and this situation is discussed further in Chapter 8.

Anxiety is also common in patients with heart failure, and may exacerbate the symptoms – especially feelings of breathlessness. There is some evidence that certain forms of relaxation therapy, including progressive muscle relaxation and meditation, can improve psychological distress and quality of life in older heart failure patients [23, 24], although effects on exercise capacity are less clear.

References

1. Witham, M.D., Struthers, A.D. and McMurdo, M.E. (2003) Exercise training as a therapy for chronic heart failure: can older people benefit? *Journal of the American Geriatrics Society*, **51**, 699–709.
2. Piepoli, M.F., Davos, C., Francis, D.P. and Coats, A.J. (2004) Exercise training meta-analysis of trials in patients with chronic heart failure (ExTraMATCH). *British Medical Journal*, **328**, 189.
3. Porcari, J.P., Foster, C., Dehar-Beverley, M. *et al.* (2004) Relationship between the talk test and ventilatory threshold. *European Journal of Cardiovascular Prevention and Rehabilitation*, **11** (Suppl 1), 57.

4. Austin, J., Williams, R., Ross, L. *et al.* (2005) Randomised controlled trial of cardiac rehabilitation in elderly patients with heart failure. *European Journal of Heart Failure*, 7, 411–417.

5. Witham, M.D., Gray, J.M., Argo, I.S. *et al.* (2005) Effect of a seated exercise program to improve physical function and health status in frail patients ≥70 years of age with heart failure. *American Journal of Cardiology*, **95**, 1120–1124.

6. Rasinaho, M., Hirvensalo, M., Leinonen, R. *et al.* (2007) Motives for and barriers to physical activity among older adults with mobility limitations. *Journal of Aging and Physical Activity*, **15**, 90–102.

7. Crombie, I.K., Irvine, L., Williams, B. *et al.* (2004) Why older people do not participate in leisure time physical activity: a survey of activity levels, beliefs and deterrents. *Age and Ageing*, **33**, 287–292.

8. Meyer, K., Schwaibold, M., Westbrook, S. *et al.* (1996) Effects of short-term exercise training and activity restriction on functional capacity in patients with severe chronic congestive heart failure. *American Journal of Cardiology*, **78**, 1017–1022.

9. Harris, S., LeMaitre, J.P., Mackenzie, G. *et al.* (2003) A randomised study of home-based electrical stimulation of the legs and conventional bicycle exercise training for patients with chronic heart failure. *European Heart Journal*, **24**, 871–878.

10. Dall'Ago, P., Chiappa, G.R., Guths, H. *et al.* (2006) Inspiratory muscle training in patients with heart failure and inspiratory muscle weakness: a randomized trial. *Journal of the American College of Cardiology*, **47**, 757–763.

11. Weiner, P., Waizman, J., Magadle, R. *et al.* (1999) The effect of specific inspiratory muscle training on the sensation of dyspnea and exercise tolerance in patients with congestive heart failure. *Clinical Cardiology*, **22**, 727–732.

12. Suskin, N., Sheth, T., Negassa, A. and Yusuf, S. (2001) Relationship of current and past smoking to mortality and morbidity in patients with left ventricular dysfunction. *Journal of the American College of Cardiology*, **37**, 1677–1682.

13. Nieminen, M.S., Harjola, V.P., Hochadel, M. *et al.* (2008) Gender related differences in patients presenting with acute heart failure. Results from EuroHeart Failure Survey II. *European Journal of Heart Failure*, **10**, 140–148.

14. Colin, R.E., Castillo, M.L., Orea, T.A. *et al.* (2004) Effects of a nutritional intervention on body composition, clinical status, and quality of life in patients with heart failure. *Nutrition*, **20**, 890–895.

15. Price, R.J., Witham, M.D. and McMurdo, M.E. (2007) Defining the nutritional status and dietary intake of older heart failure patients. *European Journal of Cardiovascular Nursing*, **6**, 178–183.

16. Gustafsson, F., Kragelund, C.B., Torp-Pedersen, C. *et al.* (2005) Effect of obesity and being overweight on long-term mortality in congestive heart failure: influence of left ventricular systolic function. *European Heart Journal*, **26**, 58–64.

17. Hanninen, S.A., Darling, P.B., Sole, M.J. *et al.* (2006) The prevalence of thiamin deficiency in hospitalized patients with congestive heart failure. *Journal of the American College of Cardiology*, **47**, 354–361.

18. Zittermann, A., Schleithoff, S.S., Tenderich, G. *et al.* (2003) Low vitamin D status: a contributing factor in the pathogenesis of congestive heart failure? *Journal of the American College of Cardiology*, **41**, 105–112.

19. Witte, K.K., Nikitin, N.P., Parker, A.C. *et al.* (2005) The effect of micronutrient supplementation on quality-of-life and left ventricular function in elderly patients with chronic heart failure. *European Heart Journal*, **26**, 2238–2244.

20. Sander, S., Coleman, C.I., Patel, A.A. *et al.* (2006) The impact of coenzyme Q10 on systolic function in patients with chronic heart failure. *Journal of Cardiac Failure*, **12**, 464–472.

21. Nichol, K.L., Margolis, K.L., Wuorenma, J. and Von Sternberg, T. (1994) The efficacy and cost effectiveness of vaccination against influenza among elderly persons living in the community. *The New England Journal of Medicine*, **331**, 778–784.

22. Lane, D.A., Chong, A.Y. and Lip, G.Y. (2005) Psychological interventions for depression in heart failure. *Cochrane Database of Systematic Reviews*, CD003329.

23. Curiati, J.A., Bocchi, E., Freire, J.O. *et al.* (2005) Meditation reduces sympathetic activation and improves the quality of life in elderly patients with optimally treated heart failure: a prospective randomized study. *Journal of Alternative and Complementary Medicine*, **11**, 465–472.

24. Yu, D.S., Lee, D.T., Woo, J. and Hui, E. (2007) Non-pharmacological interventions in older people with heart failure: effects of exercise training and relaxation therapy. *Gerontology*, **53**, 74–81.

8
Comorbidity

Andrew Elder

Western General Hospital, Crewe Road, Edinburgh

Key messages

- Multiple comorbidities are the norm in older heart failure patients.

- Comorbid diseases alter the presentation, prognosis, diagnosis and management of heart failure patients.

- Comorbid diseases which are known to be common in heart failure patients should be sought and treated optimally.

- The goals of heart failure treatment may need to be modified in the light of competing treatment agendas from comorbid disease.

8.1 Introduction

The practice of clinical medicine in older people is the management of multiple morbidities. In some patients, a single condition – for example heart failure – appears to dominate the clinical presentation, the patient's quality of life and prognosis. However, in this situation clinicians must ensure not only that the dominant condition is optimally managed, but also that the impact of other coexistent conditions – the comorbidities – is not overlooked, particularly if disease-specific guidelines or models of care are used to structure management.

In many other patients however – and particularly those aged over 85 years – no single pathology, disease or condition dominates the clinical picture. Such patients

---

A Practical Guide to Heart Failure in Older People, Edited by C Ward and M D Witham
© 2009 John Wiley & Sons, Ltd

suffer from *multimorbidity* and the classical geriatric syndromes of falls, incontinence, dementia and the frailty syndrome, each of which requires a distinct approach to clinical assessment and care.

The interaction between heart failure, comorbidity and treatment is complex. A summary of such interactions is shown in Table 8.1.

Table 8.1 Examples of interactions between heart failure and noncardiac comorbidity.

Interaction	Examples
Comorbidity worsens the symptoms, or functional impact of heart failure, or vice versa	Arthritis COPD Anaemia CKD Cognitive impairment Malnutrition
Comorbidity worsens the prognosis of heart failure	CKD [28] COPD [45] Diabetes [38] Low body weight Depression [52] Dementia Sleep-disordered breathing ? Anaemia [13] Stroke
Comorbidity complicates diagnosis	Dementia (History) COPD (clinical features, elevated BNP, echocardiography may be difficult) CKD (elevated BNP)
Treatment of comorbidity worsens heart failure	Non-steroidal anti-inflammatory drugs in arthritis ? Thiazolidinediones in diabetes TNF inhibitors in arthritis
Treatment of heart failure worsens a comorbidity	Diuretics and urinary incontinence Drugs causing postural hypotension and falls ACE inhibitors and chronic kidney disease ? Beta-blockers during exacerbations of COPD Diuretics and gout
Comorbidity complicates management	Dementia (adherence) Polypharmacy and adherence CKD (dose adjustment needed for some medicines) Reversible airways obstruction and beta-blockade

Note: Not all the studies on which these associations are based investigated exclusively elderly populations.

8.2 The prevalence of comorbidities

In a large North American study of over 120 000 patients with heart failure, all aged over 65 years and with a mean age of 80 years, only 4% had no significant noncardiac comorbid conditions. More than half of the group had four or more noncardiac comorbidities, and 4% had ten or more [1]. A number of similar studies have identified a relatively consistent pattern of cardiac and noncardiac comorbidity in older heart failure patients (see Table 8.2). Although noncardiac comorbidities are more common than cardiac comorbidities in the over 85s [2], the relative contribution of these two subsets of comorbidities to symptoms and outlook, and the frequency with which they complicate clinical management in older people, have not been formally assessed. In this chapter we focus on noncardiac comorbidity.

Table 8.2 Prevalence of the more common comorbidities in older patients with heart failure.

Noncardiac comorbidity	Estimated prevalence (%)
Chronic lung disease, particularly COPD	30
Chronic kidney disease	30–60
Anaemia	18–60
Arthritis, particularly osteoarthritis	3–16
Stroke disease	5–15
Sleep-disordered breathing	10–70
Cognitive impairment	12–50
Diabetes mellitus	30–40
Dyslipidaemia	50
Urinary incontinence	5
Gout	5
Frailty syndrome	5–10
Hyperuricaemia	20
Orthostatic hypotension	20–30
Benign prostatic hypertrophy	7
Osteoporosis	5
Peripheral vascular disease	16
Depression	13–77

Note: Not all the studies on which these figures are based investigate exclusively elderly populations. For further information, see the relevant subsection.

8.3 The implications of comorbidity

Clinical assessment and diagnosis

A common feature of the clinical assessment of older people is the presence of 'coincidental' findings in both history and physical examination that may or may not have relevance to the patient's presenting clinical condition. Clinicians should not overlook such findings, but rather consider their relevance to the patient's clinical condition, and whether they require further evaluation or management.

The difficulties of diagnosing heart failure in older patients with multiple comorbidities are well recognized (see below and Chapter 5), but have not been systematically evaluated.

Assessment of functional limitation

The use of single-symptom or disease-specific scores such as the New York Heart Association (NYHA) score, is often of limited value in older patients because of impaired mobility resulting from comorbidities. More generic assessment tools such as the Elderly Mobility Score (EMS) [3] or the Barthel Activities of Daily Living Index [4] are more relevant and valuable in day-to-day clinical practice.

Evidence base, guidelines and goals of treatment

Older patients, particularly those with comorbidities, are under-represented in the major trials of heart failure treatment (as discussed in Chapter 6). Despite a consensus that heart failure management in older patients should nevertheless follow the principles defined in these trials, evidence-based drug treatment remains under-prescribed. This probably reflects concerns about adverse effects of treatment in those with comorbidity, as well as physician scepticism regarding potential benefit [5]. Yet, even with optimal medication, improvement is more limited than in trial populations, perhaps because of the effects of inadequately addressed comorbidities [6].

Treatment goals vary from patient to patient, and few generalizations can be made. However, as age and comorbidities advance, and the average anticipated life span declines, individual patients may have varying views regarding cardiopulmonary resuscitation, and on the emphasis placed on the use of drugs designed to improve symptoms, prognosis, or both, as opposed to on the adoption of a palliative, rather than curative, model of care [7].

Drug treatment and polypharmacy

Older patients with heart failure take an average of seven different drugs each day, and those with multiple comorbidities often take more. Such polypharmacy is associated with an increased frequency of adverse events, decreased treatment adherence and increased rates of hospitalization and mortality [8].

The routine, careful and systematic review of drug treatment of older people with heart failure is therefore a critical part of care [9], and a structured medication review can improve patient outcomes when it forms part of a care management programme

[10, 11]. All clinicians should have sufficient knowledge of the indications, interactions, risks and benefits of medications prescribed for the common comorbidities of older heart failure patients. Some common problems relating to prescribing for older patients with heart failure are summarized in Table 8.3.

Models of care

Older patients with heart failure are currently cared for by a variety of primary and secondary care teams. For example, in a large Medicare population only 10% of the patients were cared for by cardiologists, 50% by generalists, and the remainder by other organ specialists [1]. Although it has been suggested that specialist cardiology care might improve heart failure-related prescribing and outcomes, that idea has not been formally assessed in any trial setting. There is, however, no objective evidence that older heart failure patients with multimorbidity who are cared for by cardiologists have better outcomes than those cared for by other physicians.

Currently, Comprehensive Geriatric Assessment (CGA) – that is, the assessment by a specialist geriatrician and multidisciplinary team, covering all aspects of physical, cognitive, psychological and social function – provides an established evidence-based model [12] to approach the care of patients with multimorbidity. This approach identifies comorbidity effectively, and targets treatment and rehabilitation at patient-centred holistic outcomes of function, independence and health rather than disease-specific outcomes or mortality alone. Ideally, all older patients with heart failure and multimorbidity should have access to such structured care. If not, they should be screened for significant comorbidity by a clinician with experience in the assessment and management of multimorbidity.

8.4 Specific comorbidities in heart failure

Anaemia

Prevalence

Estimates of the prevalence of anaemia in heart failure vary widely according to the precise population studied and the definition of anaemia used [13,14], but can range between 20% and 60%. The prevalence is higher in patients who are older, have associated chronic kidney disease (CKD), and more advanced heart failure.

Aetiology

Haemodilution is imprecisely defined in many studies, but is a common causative or contributory factor in anaemia [15]. A minority of patients have either microcytic (typically iron-deficient) or macrocytic (typically relating to folate or vitamin B_{12}

Table 8.3   Examples of interactions between drug therapy, comorbidity and heart failure in older patients.

Comorbidity	Drug	Interaction with heart failure
Orthostatic hypotension	Fludrocortisone	Fluid retention
Benign prostatic hypertrophy	Alpha-blockers	Exacerbate tendency to postural hypotension in those on heart failure drugs.
COPD	Long-acting beta$_2$ agonists	? Increased incidence of adverse cardiac outcomes
Dementia	Acetylcholinesterase inhibitors	May exacerbate bradycardia
Diabetes mellitus	Thiazolidinediones	Fluid retention
	Metformin	? Increased risk of lactic acidosis
Rheumatoid arthritis	NSAIDs Glucocorticoids TNF inhibitors	May exacerbate heart failure
Anaemia	Blood transfusion	Volume overload and worsening heart failure
Osteoarthritis	NSAIDs/COX-II inhibitors	Fluid retention; renal dysfunction
Chronic kidney disease		Attenuated diuretic effect Increased risk of intolerance of ACE inhibitors Digoxin dose modification
Osteoarthritis	Non-steroidal anti-inflammatory drugs	Fluid retention
		Renal dysfunction
		Interaction with other comorbidity
Heart failure		
	Loop diuretic	May impair continence May provoke delirium secondary to metabolic upset Reduces bone mineral density May provoke gout
	Thiazide diuretic	May impair continence Increases bone mineral density
	Potassium-sparing diuretics	Increased risk of hyperkalaemia in CKD
	ACE inhibitors	May worsen renal function and provoke delirium May impair continence (cough)
	Angiotensin-receptor blockers	May worsen renal function and provoke delirium
	Beta-blockers	? Tolerability in patients with exacerbations of COPD
	Digoxin	? Enhanced risk of delirium in those with pre-existing cognitive impairment

deficiency) anaemias. The majority of anaemias are normocytic, sometimes attributable to CKD, but most commonly to heart failure *per se* via several mechanisms, most prominently elevated serum levels of proinflammatory cytokines.

Prognosis

Anaemia may have an adverse effect on the progression and severity of heart failure [13]. When anaemia is severe there may be salt and water retention, a reduction of the estimated glomerular filtration rate (eGFR), and activation of the renin-angiotensin-aldosterone system [16]. In less severe cases, a reduced oxygen delivery to the skeletal muscle can contribute to an impaired exercise capacity [17]. Some observational studies support the concept that reduced haemoglobin levels are associated with poorer outcomes [18,19], although in the largest study – in which confounding factors were analyzed in detail – there was no suggestion of any independent effect of anaemia on prognosis in patients with heart failure [20].

Investigation

The basic approach to the investigation and treatment of anaemia should be similar in older patients, with and without underlying heart failure [21].

Treatment

If a patient with heart failure becomes anaemic, the reversible underlying causes should be identified and treated appropriately. Parenteral iron may be required if oral preparations cannot be tolerated or absorbed.

A variety of additional strategies may be employed in patients in whom anaemia is thought to be relate to heart failure, or to heart failure and CKD in combination. Intravenous iron has been shown, in small studies, to improve exercise capacity and reduce B-type natriuretic peptide (BNP) levels, even in patients without any clear evidence of iron deficiency [22, 23]. Further evaluation of such treatment is required before its extended use is promoted.

Although erythropoietin levels are elevated in anaemic patients with heart failure, the levels are less than expected for the degree of anaemia observed. Erythropoietic agents such as recombinant human erythropoietin have therefore been evaluated [24]. Although symptomatic and prognostic benefits have been reported, concern persists about adverse effects (e.g. a prothrombotic effect) [13,25] and the small patient numbers of many studies. The results of the most recent and largest study conducted to date demonstrated neither significant clinical benefit nor significant adverse effects [26]. However, some patients with heart failure, moderate to severe CKD and haemoglobin levels less than 11 g dl^{-1} may derive symptomatic benefit, and careful use of erythropoietin should be considered in this group [13].

Blood transfusion should be considered if the haemoglobin level is less than $7\,\mathrm{g\,dl}^{-1}$ (the level below which adverse haemodynamic consequences can be demonstrated), particularly if the patient is symptomatic and there is no correctible haematinic deficiency. In patients with acute myocardial infarction, many of whom have new or established impairment of left ventricular (LV) function, a blood transfusion will have a prognostic benefit if the haematocrit is below 30% [27].

Chronic kidney disease (CKD)

Chronic kidney disease and heart failure are closely interrelated. Both conditions are common in older people, who are therefore more likely than younger patients to suffer from the recognized adverse effects on renal function of standard medications, and of disturbances in fluid balance. This means that the optimization of treatment is more difficult, or even impossible, to achieve.

Definition and prevalence

Today, the clinical assessment of renal function should be routinely based on the calculation of eGFR rather than measurement of serum creatinine alone, as this provides a more reliable measurement, particularly in older age. Online tools exist to facilitate calculation and to classify the degree of renal dysfunction into the five stages of CKD. Renal dysfunction is likely to be of potential clinical significance in older heart failure patients at eGFR values $<60\,\mathrm{ml\,min}^{-1}$ (stage 3, 4, 5 CKD), but milder degrees of dysfunction should not be disregarded.

In a recent meta-analysis, 63% of heart failure patients (mean age 73 years) were found to have renal impairment (eGFR $<90\,\mathrm{ml\,min}^{-1}$) which was moderate to severe (eGFR $<53\,\mathrm{ml\,min}^{-1}$) in 29% [28]. Adjusted all-cause mortality was doubled in those with moderate to severe renal impairment compared to those with normal renal function. The extent that renal dysfunction itself contributes to the excess mortality, as opposed to the effect of underutilization of effective treatments in patients with renal dysfunction, remains uncertain.

Aetiology

The presence of primary disease of either the heart or kidney can lead to secondary dysfunction of the other organ. Patients with primary renal disease have an increased incidence of heart failure secondary to hypertension, fluid retention, and accelerated atherosclerotic disease. Patients with congestive heart failure (CHF) may also develop renal dysfunction in the absence of intrinsic renal disease, as a direct consequence of heart failure in itself. This relates to a decreasing cardiac output and a resultant decrease in renal perfusion, with intrarenal vasoconstriction and consequent salt and water retention.

The aetiology of CKD in heart failure patients is diverse, and should not be assumed to relate to heart failure or drug treatment of heart failure alone.

- In all older patients presenting with new or deteriorating renal function, the possibility of intrinsic renal disease, particularly due to noncardiovascular drug treatment or obstructive uropathy, should be considered.

- Intercurrent illness of any sort in frail, older patients may result in a decline in fluid intake or an increase in nonurinary fluid loss, leading in turn to intravascular volume depletion and prerenal uraemia.

- The finding of prerenal uraemia should not therefore be assumed to relate to diuretic treatment alone. Older patients with heart failure and newly identified renal dysfunction should undergo urinalysis, renal and bladder ultrasonography, a careful drug review and a clinical assessment of volume status and fluid intake, output and balance.

The treatment of intercurrent urinary infection, the withdrawal of nephrotoxic drugs and the relief of any prostatic obstruction can, in particular, result in a significant improvement of impaired renal function.

But, how does the presence of renal dysfunction influence the efficacy and safety of drug treatment for heart failure?

The efficacy and safety of standard treatment for heart failure is less certain in patients with CKD, as many of the major drug trials have specifically excluded patients with renal dysfunction, and notably those who are older. In general, the presence of CKD implies a potentially attenuated therapeutic response to diuretics and an increased risk of toxicity from ACE inhibitors, angiotensin-receptor blockers, digoxin, aldosterone antagonists and water-soluble beta-blockers. In addition, any heart failure treatments that may cause hypotension through any mechanism, including intravascular volume depletion, may also worsen renal dysfunction.

ACE inhibitors

In the few studies which included significant numbers of patients with moderate renal dysfunction (eGFR 30–60 ml min^{-1}) the limited evidence supports efficacy of a similar level to that found in patients with normal renal function [29]. Many authorities recommend avoiding ACE inhibitors in patients with severe renal dysfunction (eGFR <30 ml min^{-1}), or using them only with extreme caution. In clinical practice, in older patients with eGFR <60 ml min^{-1}, clinicians should commence with small doses and any up-titration should be gradual, being based on symptomatic effect and tolerance and not on a 'prognostic' dose target. Serum creatinine and potassium levels should also be closely monitored. The management of deteriorating renal function following the introduction of ACE inhibitors is described below. The general approach to the use of angiotensin-receptor blockers should be similar to that outlined for ACE inhibitors.

Other vasodilators

The combination of hydralazine and isosorbide mononitrate has prognostic benefit in heart failure [30], and may be tolerated in older patients with renal dysfunction who cannot tolerate ACE inhibitors or angiotensin-receptor blockers.

Beta-blockers

Most large clinical trials of beta-blockers have excluded patients with varying degrees of renal dysfunction [31]. The exception was the CIBIS II trial [32], in which a subgroup of patients with renal dysfunction reported similar outcomes to those without renal dysfunction. The available evidence therefore suggests that a 'start low–go slow' approach to dosing and titration would be reasonable.

Spironolactone

Although the efficacy and safety of spironolactone appeared similar across the range of renal function included in the RALES analysis [33], the proportion of patients studied with severe renal insufficiency appears to have been small. Subsequent case series have implicated renal dysfunction as a risk factor for hyperkalaemia in older patients [34]. Spironolactone should therefore be avoided if the eGFR is <30 ml min^{-1}, while in patients with milder degrees of renal dysfunction care should be taken to monitor serum potassium levels very closely.

Diuretics

There are a number of reasons for abnormal salt and water homeostasis in older, more frail patients. It is therefore clinically prudent to commence treatment with standard doses (20–40 mg furosemide) in this patient subgroup, whilst recognizing that in the presence of renal dysfunction, much higher doses (single doses of $\geq$120 mg intravenous furosemide, $\geq$5 mg oral bumetanide, or $\geq$40 mg torasemide) may be necessary to achieve maximal diuresis. As with all prescribing in older people, the procedure is to 'start low' and 'go slow'.

Digoxin

As digoxin is cleared by the kidney, renal dysfunction will increase the likelihood of digoxin toxicity and necessitate maintenance dose reduction. In the largest study of digoxin use in heart failure patients [35], those with a serum creatinine >265 μmol l^{-1}

were excluded, and no analysis of effect according to the level of renal dysfunction was published. If digoxin is indicated in a patient in sinus rhythm with heart failure and renal dysfunction, or in atrial fibrillation when rapid rate control is not indicated, then digoxin can be effectively and safely introduced, without a loading dose.

How should deteriorating renal function in a patient with known heart failure be approached?

Prerenal uraemia caused by the treatment of heart failure is common in older heart failure patients, often due to a combination of over-diuresis and hypoperfusion due to vasodilator therapy. When drug treatment for heart failure is the suspected cause, a recent drug history should be taken to identify potential culprit drugs; these should be withdrawn sequentially with regular monitoring of renal function.

Having excluded causes not directly related to treatment:

- Particular attention should be paid to the maintenance of adequate oral fluid intake, especially in more frail patients.

- If renal dysfunction is severe, or marked intravascular volume depletion or hypotension is present, all possibly implicated drugs may need to be withdrawn immediately.

Minimizing the likelihood of significant renal dysfunction in older heart failure patients

Renal function is more likely to decline at the time of introduction of ACE inhibitors if patients are taking larger doses of diuretics, or are in negative fluid balance. A careful clinical assessment of fluid and volume status should therefore be made before ACE inhibitor introduction. The possibility of renal dysfunction developing after the introduction of ACE inhibition is also greatly increased by the coincident prescription of NSAIDs, and this combination should be avoided in older patients.

Patients hospitalized with heart failure, or undergoing any up-titration of diuretic dose at home, should be closely monitored for evidence of over-diuresis or intravascular volume depletion. Measurements of serum urea and the recording of daily body weights will help to ensure that over-diuresis does not occur. Many clinicians recommend a target weight loss of no more than 0.5–1 kg per day in older oedematous patients, although some may tolerate a more rapid diuresis.

Diabetes mellitus

Diabetes occurs in approximately 30–40% of older patients with heart failure [1]. Diabetic patients have an increased incidence of cardiovascular disease, including coronary artery disease (CAD), hypertension and heart failure. Heart failure may develop as a consequence of the associated CAD or hypertension, but also occurs independently of these conditions; a specific diabetic cardiomyopathy is recognized. In published studies, the overall relative risk ratio for the development of heart failure in patients with diabetes mellitus is 2.4–5 [36].

The prevalence of heart failure and associated hospitalization is higher in patients with less well-controlled diabetes [37], and heart failure patients with coexistent diabetes have a higher mortality than those without [38].

Clinical implications

The management of heart failure should follow the same principles as in patients without diabetes, and limited evidence from subgroup analysis in heart failure trials suggests similar outcomes. Weight loss is recommended for diabetic patients who are obese, and this may improve exercise capacity in patients with CHF.

ACE inhibitors have specific benefits in patients with heart failure and diabetes by limiting the progression of diabetic nephropathy and retinopathy, and by aiding blood pressure control. In addition, losartan has been shown to reduce the incidence of first hospitalization for new heart failure in diabetic patients [37].

Given the association between poorer diabetic control and prognosis, there is interest in the effects of different treatments for diabetes on heart failure outcomes [39]. An increased risk of lactic acidosis in heart failure patients, particularly in the presence of renal dysfunction, has been associated with metformin, although both meta-analysis [40] and observational studies [41] suggest that the risk is low and mortality in diabetic patients with heart failure may actually be lower when treated with metformin. Although information on the specific effects of sulfonylureas and insulin is less conclusive, there is no reason to modify the use of these treatments in patients with heart failure and diabetes.

Thiazolidinediones (glitazones) may cause fluid retention and are associated with an increased risk of developing heart failure [42]. They are, therefore, currently contraindicated in heart failure.

Chronic obstructive pulmonary disease (COPD)

Prevalence, prognosis and common features

As many as one-third of patients with heart failure have associated COPD [43], which is an independent risk factor for the development of cardiovascular disease, including heart failure [44]. The prognosis is worse when the two conditions coexist, as patients with heart failure and COPD are over fivefold more likely to be hospitalized than patients with heart failure alone [45]. Both conditions not only cause breathlessness, but also produce a catabolic state and cause skeletal myopathy, further limiting exercise capacity [43].

Clinical implications

Diagnosis

- Breathlessness is a cardinal symptom of both heart failure and COPD.

- Orthopnoea, peripheral oedema, cough, resting tachycardia, an elevated jugular venous pressure, a gallop rhythm, wheeze or prolonged expiration may occur in both conditions.

- In the absence of an infective exacerbation, signs of hyperinflation may be the only evidence of the presence of COPD.

- Clinicians must have a high level of suspicion of the presence of heart failure in COPD patients, and vice versa.

This topic is also discussed in Chapter 5.

Investigation

Specific features of either condition may be apparent on chest radiography, but have low sensitivity. Arterial blood gas analysis, cardiopulmonary exercise testing and pulmonary function testing show no specific patterns that indicate the coexistence of heart failure and COPD. In addition, deconditioning, frailty and an inability to undertake pulmonary function or exercise testing in very old or cognitively impaired individuals, further limits the diagnostic utility of such investigations.

Clinicians should adopt a critical approach to the aetiology of exercise limitation, dyspnoea and peripheral oedema in patients with known heart failure, who have an apparently suboptimal response to tailored therapy. Evidence of hyperinflation should be sought, and a smoking history ascertained. Pulmonary function testing may provide supporting evidence of airways obstruction, but even when this is absent a trial of COPD treatment in patients with a suboptimal response to optimal heart failure treatment may be appropriate.

Specific issues of COPD management include:

- Cough is no more common with the use of ACE inhibitors in patients with heart failure and COPD than in those with heart failure alone [46].

- Evidence for the use of beta-blockers in patients with COPD is discussed in Chapter 6; COPD is not an automatic contraindication to their use.

- Graded exercise programmes may confer additional benefit in selected patients with COPD alone or heart failure alone, and although no evidence exists to assess benefit in patients with concurrent heart failure and COPD, there is no reason to suggest that selected patients cannot benefit to a similar degree.

Cognitive impairment

Dementia

Dementia is a chronic progressive neurological disorder characterized by impairment of memory and at least one other cognitive domain, such as executive functioning. Alzheimer's disease and vascular dementia are the most commonly identified forms. Dementia affects 30–45% of patients aged over 85 years, and the prevalence is set to double over the next 20 years.

Delirium

Delirium (or acute confusional state or acute brain failure) is a clinical syndrome characterized by disturbances of consciousness, perception and cognition to varying degrees, usually in the context of an identifiable precipitant. As many as 30% of older patients experience delirium during hospital admission, and it is associated with a longer length of stay and poorer health outcomes [47].

Prevalence and impact on prognosis

Several studies focussing primarily on dementia rather than delirium have shown that cognitive impairment is more common in patients with heart failure than in age-matched controls (risk ratio 1.5–1.8, prevalence 12–50%), depending on the population studied [48]. The combination is associated with a higher mortality and increased functional dependence in activities of daily living than is found in matched patients with heart failure alone.

The coexistence of the two conditions may be coincidental, but in some it may be partly related to the presence of shared risk factors, particularly atrial fibrillation, hypertension and diabetes mellitus. There is also speculation that heart failure may lead more directly to the development of cognitive dysfunction due to hypotension and chronic cerebral hypoperfusion caused by reduced cardiac output or the use of vasodilating drugs [49].

Clinical implications

Clearly, patients with cognitive impairment may not present their symptoms in the same way as non-impaired heart failure patients; a heightened level of diagnostic suspicion is therefore necessary. Observations from carers regarding decline in functional capacity, sleep disturbance or progressive oedema may be useful.

The routine screening of older patients with tools such as the 30-point Mini Mental State Examination (MMSE) is useful, and because depression can cause diagnostic confusion, a psychiatric review should be considered in cases of uncertainty. Centrally acting cholinesterase inhibitors [50] (e.g. donepezil, rivastigmine, galantamine) are increasingly used in the treatment of dementia, but should be administered with caution to patients with sick-sinus syndrome, bradycardia or with conduction abnormalities. Such agents may also worsen delirium in an acute setting. Patients with heart failure and dementia may require more professional and carer supervision or support in order to adhere to drug treatment, diet or self-management programmes (as discussed in Chapter 7).

Delirium may precipitate admission to hospital and complicate the management of heart failure. Intravascular volume depletion, with prerenal uraemia, sustained hypotension and hypoperfusion due to heart failure itself or associated drug treatment, and electrolyte abnormalities such as hyponatraemia, hypokalaemia and hypomagnesaemia, may cause such reversible confusion. Occasionally, lipid-soluble beta-blockers or digoxin may cause delirium or other neuropsychiatric side effects.

All inpatient units treating older heart failure patients should recognize the high prevalence of dementia, and have established protocols for the screening, diagnosis (ideally using standardized tools such as the CAM score [51]) and identification of correctible underlying causes, as well as providing treatment and carer education and reassurance.

Depression

Depression is common, affects patients of all ages, and is particularly common in those with coexistent physical illness, including cardiovascular disease. It may coexist with anxiety states and cognitive impairment in the old, complicating diagnosis and management, and increasing evidence suggests that it is both under-diagnosed and under-treated in patients with heart failure [52]. The overall prevalence is about 20%, but this is likely to be higher in patients hospitalized for heart failure.

Depression may be an independent risk factor for the development of a variety of cardiovascular conditions, including heart failure [52], and mortality is increased if the depression is moderate or severe. For treatment, selective serotonin reuptake inhibitors (SSRIs) are preferred to tricyclic antidepressants because of the relatively high incidence of cardiac adverse effects with the latter agents.

Stroke

It is estimated that 5–10% of patients with heart failure have suffered from a stroke [1, 53], although specific research in large populations of older heart failure patients is surprisingly limited. Clearly, the coexistence of stroke may modify the clinical presentation and functional limitation of heart failure, particularly if communication or mobility are already restricted, but the general approach to investigation and management should not be altered.

Chronic heart failure is a risk factor for stroke, with the risk increasing further in the presence of atrial fibrillation, LV thrombus formation and severity of LV systolic dysfunction. In clinical practice, given the shared risk factors and overlap in the incidence of these two conditions, the routine assessment of LV function by echocardiography is logical in patients with stroke.

In patients with atrial fibrillation, anticoagulation is effective and should be prescribed unless absolute contraindications exist, the patient declines such therapy, or the level of frailty and limited life expectancy imposed by multimorbidity is likely to nullify the potential benefit. Current guidelines do not recommend the routine use of warfarin in heart failure in sinus rhythm, although the results of further specific trials are awaited; patients with LV thrombus or aneurysm may however benefit from warfarin, even when in sinus rhythm [54]. If not receiving warfarin, aspirin is generally recommended in patients with heart failure, despite limited evidence from prospective trials specifically investigating its safety and efficacy.

Falls

Falls are highly prevalent in all countries with ageing populations, and are more likely to occur in older patients and in those with multiple comorbidities. Falls are under-reported by patients, under-diagnosed by clinicians, associated with negative health outcomes and often, erroneously, assumed to be part of normal ageing and not amenable to prevention. Approximately 30% of people aged over 65 years and 50% aged over 80 years will fall each year [55], and such events are associated with increased fracture rates, emergency attendances at hospital, hospital bed utilization, decreased functional capacity and quality of life and the loss of independent living [56].

No direct link between heart failure and falls has been identified, but patients with heart failure suffer from impaired autonomic vascular tone, are receiving multiple drugs associated with falls and urinary incontinence, and suffer from muscle weakness – all risk factors for falls. Patients with multiple comorbid conditions and polypharmacy are at more risk of falling [57], and as these are common features of the older heart failure population, such patients should be regarded as being at high risk of falls.

Interventions for falls are based on multifactorial risk reduction, and evidence exists to suggest efficacy for a variety of such strategies [58]. In addition, calcium and vitamin D supplementation reduces falls and fractures in institutionalized older people [59]. There is also limited evidence that targeted drug review and withdrawal if possible – including diuretics and, more surprisingly, digoxin – may reduce fall frequency [60].

In routine clinical practice, all clinicians encountering older heart failure patients should adopt a simple three-point approach:

- All older patients should be asked at least once each year about falls.

- All older patients who report a single fall should be observed performing the 'Get Up and Go' test [61]. Further assessment is necessary if patients have difficulty or demonstrate unsteadiness while performing this test.

- Older patients who present for medical attention because of a fall or who report recurrent falls in the past year should have a fall evaluation performed. This may necessitate referral to a specialist (e.g. a geriatrician) if the primary provider is not experienced in this evaluation.

Orthostatic hypotension

Evidence linking drug treatment in heart failure with postural hypotension is conflicting [62], but in clinical practice it is frequently observed – and, more importantly, symptoms improve – following drug withdrawal in patients taking diuretics, ACE inhibitors, angiotensin-receptor blockers or beta-blockers. Possible causative mechanisms include intravascular volume depletion, impaired heart rate responsiveness to an upright posture, vasodilation and sustained supine hypotension. Less commonly, hypoadrenalism or autonomic neuropathy underlie the problem, especially if severe.

In patients in whom heart failure medication is felt to be implicated, intravascular volume status should be carefully assessed, followed by judicious salt and water replacement, if necessary. A subsequent careful down-titration or cessation of relevant drugs, or a relaxation of salt or fluid restriction, is then necessary in an attempt to find a compromise between heart failure treatment doses that control symptoms without causing limiting symptomatic hypotension.

Standard treatments for postural hypotension (fludrocortisone, NSAIDs, midodrine, erythropoietin, non-selective beta-blockers or support stockings) are either contraindicated or have not been fully assessed in heart failure. In practice, most benefit appears to result from drug review and down-titration or withdrawal, plus simple patient advice and education.

Arthritis

Older patients with heart failure frequently have a coexistent arthropathy, typically relating to large joint osteoarthritis (OA), and less commonly due to chronic rheumatoid arthritis (RA).

Prevalence

The prevalence of OA is 16%, and of RA is approximately 3% [1]. Although there is no direct aetiological link between OA and heart failure, such a link has been

identified with RA, and this may contribute to an increased mortality in these
patients [63].

The aetiological link with RA may be due to high circulating levels of inflammatory mediators, previous or concurrent use of drug treatment for RA, including
glucocorticoids and tumour necrosis factor (TNF) inhibitors, and a higher prevalence of CAD and of amyloidosis.

Clinical implications

Functionally limiting arthropathy may lead to a delayed or incorrect diagnosis of
heart failure in immobile patients, peripheral oedema may be caused by hypoalbu-
minaemia in patients with chronic debilitating arthropathy, and the occurrence of
pulmonary crackles in a patient with RA may relate to either pulmonary fibrosis or
heart failure.

The treatment of RA and OA is more difficult in patients with heart failure: The
use of NSAIDs, and also of some cyclo-oxygenase (COX)-II inhibitors, should be
minimized or precluded, particularly in patients receiving ACE inhibitors, because of
the adverse effects of this combination on renal function. Fluid retention and an
attenuation of the effect of diuretics can also occur, even in the absence of renal
dysfunction or concurrent ACE inhibitor use. Given concerns about the deterioration of heart failure, which may precipitate hospitalization, TNF inhibitors should
also be avoided. Glucocorticoids can also exacerbate heart failure, and although not
absolutely contraindicated, careful monitoring of fluid status is needed; diuretic
doses often need to increase when introducing steroids.

Sleep-disordered breathing (SDB)

Definitions and prevalence

Obstructive sleep apnoea–hypopnoea (OSAH) and central sleep apnoea syndrome
(CSAS) are the most common forms of sleep-disordered breathing observed in
patients with congestive heart failure. In contrast to the normal population, CSAS
(as typified by Cheyne–Stokes breathing) is more common than OSAH. Sleep-
disordered breathing can contribute to the development and progression of heart
failure and prognosis is poorer in patients with heart failure and SDB, most likely
because of its detrimental haemodynamic effects and the increased frequency of
arrhythmia.

Clinical implications

Sleep-disordered breathing in heart failure may be either symptomatic or asymptomatic, and an awareness of its high prevalence is central to its recognition. A

sleep history from both patient and spouse should be taken; recurrent arrhythmias, nocturnal angina and otherwise unexplained refractory heart failure may indicate underlying SDB. An overnight polysomnogram is the 'gold standard' for diagnosis.

The effective treatment of congestive heart failure may also improve concurrent SDB [64]. Conversely, the treatment of SDB may reduce the frequency of sleep-related events, and some heart failure-related outcomes. In particular, continuous positive airway pressure (CPAP) has a variety of beneficial haemodynamic effects [65], with the 6-minute walking distance being improved in one large study [66]. There is, however, no clear evidence of any reduced mortality in patients with OSAH and heart failure, and CPAP should therefore be used primarily on symptomatic grounds.

Frailty and undernutrition

The frailty syndrome (or Failure to Thrive in the Elderly) is being increasingly recognized as a discrete clinical entity comprising poor effort tolerance, low physical activity levels, low body weight (with or without ongoing weight loss), decreased appetite, low serum cholesterol, impaired immune function, a feeling of exhaustion or fatigue, depression and cognitive impairment in varying degrees [67]. Importantly, the presence of frailty is associated with subsequent disability and death, independent of the effects of comorbid diseases, health habits and psychosocial characteristics [68].

Many features of the frailty syndrome are also recognized in advanced heart failure as cardiac cachexia. The precise contribution of heart failure, rather than comorbidity or advanced age, to this syndrome are often impossible to define, and generic approaches to management are therefore appropriate. An accumulation of oedema may mask skeletal muscle loss if weight alone is monitored, and patients or carers should be asked about appetite and fluid intake; a formal nutritional assessment may also be valuable. Poor nutrition contributes to immune deficiency, and may in part explain the increased tendency of congestive heart failure patients to develop infection; weight loss and low body weight have both been shown to be associated with poorer outcomes. Poor nutrition may be related to the effects of competing comorbidities on the ability to swallow, appetite, enjoyment of eating, or relate to social isolation or financial restriction. Simple problems such as ill-fitting dentures may be easily correctible. If salt restriction is suggested as part of the heart failure management, the implications for overall nutritional intake should be carefully considered to ensure that the protein and calories intake do not decline due to the unpalatability or unfamiliarity of alternative foodstuffs.

The recognition of frailty is critical to the good management of older patients with heart failure and multiple comorbidities, and should also prompt consideration of the overall goals of treatment, the goals of treatment of specific comorbidities, the need for coordinated comprehensive geriatric assessment, the value of limited exercise programmes, and the appropriateness of continuing preventative rather than purely symptomatic treatments.

Urinary incontinence

The prevalence and severity of urinary incontinence increases with age in both males and females, is under-recognized and under-treated, and may contribute significantly to patient-perceived poor QOL and functional limitation [69]. As a result, incontinence is one cause of the well-documented reduced adherence to treatment in heart failure [70], as diuretic therapy may worsen incontinence – particularly in those with detrusor instability or dyssenergia, when the bladder capacity is limited. Unfortunately, many patients and their clinicians may not appreciate this point, nor that it can be satisfactorily and simply managed if properly investigated. Patients may instead choose *not* to take diuretics rather than to report the problem to their doctor. All enquiries about urinary symptoms should therefore be made sensitively and routinely.

Systematic evaluation and management can improve symptoms in many older people. None of the drugs commonly used for bladder instability or prostatic hypertrophy is specifically contraindicated in heart failure, although most (e.g. anticholinergics and alpha-blockers) can worsen postural (orthostatic) hypotension. Simple explanations of the mode of action of diuretics and the usual time course of diuresis may help patients tailor their dose timings to their own activity schedule. Patients should be advised to time their diuretic doses around daily activities, for example taking a loop diuretic dose on first waking, such that diuresis is over by mid to late morning.

Although urinary catheterization is not always tolerated nor acceptable, some older and frailer patients will choose this option if offered, if it enables them to avoid troublesome frequency or unmanageable incontinence, particularly if their mobility is significantly impaired or skin care jeopardized.

Sensory deprivation

In general, sight, hearing, taste and smell all decline in older age. Each deficit should be evaluated for correctible problems, and not assumed to be irreversible, untreatable associations of ageing *per se*. When present, visual and auditory problems can in particular compromise a patient's ability to understand or adhere to treatment recommendations. Carer support should be utilized in these situations to maximize treatment understanding and adherence.

Osteoporosis

Limited evidence suggests an association between heart failure and low bone mineral density, although no direct effect of either condition on the other has been demonstrated, and the association may simply reflect shared risk factors relating to age, frailty and nutrition [71].

Treatment with combined oestrogen and progestogen [72] may increase the risk of cardiovascular disease and consequent heart failure. There is some concern that bisphosphonates may increase the incidence of atrial fibrillation, although all-cause mortality may in fact be lower with bisphosphonates; further research is necessary. Loop diuretics may cause a decline in bone mineral density and an increase in fracture rate [73], while conversely thiazide diuretics may increase bone mineral density and reduce fracture risk [74]. However, the clinical significance of these findings is uncertain, and at present older heart failure patients with concurrent osteoporosis should be managed in the standard fashion.

References

1. Braunstein, J.B., Anderson, G.F., Gerstenblith, G. *et al.* (2003) Noncardiac comorbidity increases preventable hospitalizations and mortality among Medicare beneficiaries with chronic heart failure. *Journal of the American College of Cardiology*, **42**, 1226–1233.
2. van der Wel, M.C., Jansen, R.W., Bakx, J.C. *et al.* (2007) Non-cardiovascular co-morbidity in elderly patients with heart failure outnumbers cardiovascular co-morbidity. *European Journal of Heart Failure*, **9**, 709–715.
3. Smith, R. (1994) Validation and reliability of the elderly mobility scale. *Physiotherapy*, **80**, 744–747.
4. Sinoff, G. and Ore, L. (1997) The Barthel Activities of Daily Living Index: self reporting versus actual performance in the old-old (greater than 75 years). *Journal of the American Geriatric Society*, **45** (7), 832–836.
5. Fuat, A., Pali, A., Hungin, S. and Murphy, J.J. (2003) Barriers to accurate diagnosis and effective management of heart failure in primary care: a qualitative study. *British Medical Journal*, **326**, 196–202.
6. Welch, G.H., Albertsen, P.C., Nease, R.F. *et al.* (1996) Estimating treatment benefits for the elderly: the effect of competing risks. *Annals of Internal Medicine*, **124**, 577–584.
7. Stevenson, J., Abernethy, A.P., Miller, C. and Currow, D.C. (2004) Managing comorbidities in patients at the end of life. *British Medical Journal*, **329**, 909–912.
8. Masoudi, F.A., Baillie, C.A., Wang, Y. *et al.* (2005) The complexity and cost of drug regimens of older patients hospitalized with heart failure in the United States, 1998–2001. *Archives of Internal Medicine*, **165**, 2069–2076.
9. Amabile, C.M. and Spencer, A.P. (2004) Keeping your patient with heart failure safe: a review of potentially dangerous medications. *Archives of Internal Medicine*, **164**, 709–720.
10. Rich, M.W., Beckham, V., Wittenberg, C. *et al.* (1995) A multidisciplinary intervention to prevent the readmission of elderly patients with congestive heart failure. *The New England Journal of Medicine*, **333**, 1190–1195.

11. Krumholz, H.M., Amatruda, J., Smith, G.L. *et al.* (2002) Randomized trial of an education and support intervention to prevent readmission of patients with heart failure. *Journal of the American College of Cardiology*, **39**, 83–89.

12. Stuck, A.E., Siu, A.L., Wieland, G.D. *et al.* (1993) Comprehensive geriatric assessment: a meta-analysis of controlled trials. *Lancet*, **342**, 1032–1036.

13. Tang, Y. and Katz, S.D. (2006) Anemia in chronic heart failure: prevalence, etiology, clinical correlates, and treatment options. *Circulation*, **113**, 2454–2461.

14. Cromie, N., Lee, C. and Struthers, A.D. (2002) Anaemia in chronic heart failure: what is its frequency in the UK and its underlying causes? *Heart*, **87**, 377–378.

15. Androne, A.S., Katz, S.D., Lund, L. *et al.* (2003) Hemodilution is common in patients with advanced heart failure. *Circulation*, **107**, 226–229.

16. Weiskopf, R.B., Viele, M.K., Feiner, J. *et al.* (1998) Human cardiovascular and metabolic response to acute, severe isovolemic anemia. *The Journal of the American Medical Association*, **279**, 217–221.

17. Anand, I., McMurray, J.J., Whitmore, J. *et al.* (2004) Anemia and its relationship to clinical outcome in heart failure. *Circulation*, **110**, 149–154.

18. Ezekowitz, J.A., McAlister, F.A. and Armstrong, P.W. (2003) Anemia is common in heart failure and is associated with poor outcomes: insights from a cohort of 12 065 patients with new-onset heart failure. *Circulation*, **107**, 223–225.

19. Horwich, T.B., Fonarow, G.C., Hamilton, M.A. *et al.* (2002) Anemia is associated with worse symptoms, greater impairment in functional capacity and a significant increase in mortality in patients with advanced heart failure. *Journal of the American College of Cardiology*, **39**, 1780–1786.

20. Kosiborod, M., Curtis, J.P., Wang, Y. *et al.* (2005) Anemia and outcomes in patients with heart failure: a study from the National Heart Care Project. *Archives of Internal Medicine*, **165**, 2237–2244.

21. Steensma, D.P. and Tefferi, A. (2007) Anemia in the elderly: how should we define it, when does it matter, and what can be done? *Mayo Clinic Proceedings*, **82**, 958–966.

22. Bolger, A.P., Bartlett, F.R., Penston, H.S. *et al.* (2006) Intravenous iron alone for the treatment of anemia in patients with chronic heart failure. *Journal of the American College of Cardiology*, **48**, 1225–1227.

23. Toblli, J.E., Lombrana, A., Duarte, P. and Di Gennaro, F. (2007) Intravenous iron reduces NT-pro-brain natriuretic peptide in anemic patients with chronic heart failure and renal insufficiency. *Journal of the American College of Cardiology*, **50**, 1657–1665.

24. Silverberg, D.S., Wexler, D., Blum, M. *et al.* (2000) The use of subcutaneous erythropoietin and intravenous iron for the treatment of the anemia of severe, resistant congestive heart failure improves cardiac and renal function and functional cardiac class, and markedly reduces hospitalizations. *Journal of the American College of Cardiology*, **35**, 1737–1744.

25. Felker, G.M., Adams, K.F. Jr, Gattis, W.A. and O'Connor, C.M. (2004) Anemia as a risk factor and therapeutic target in heart failure. *Journal of the American College of Cardiology*, **44**, 959–966.

26. Ghali, J.K., Anand, I.S., Abraham, W.T. *et al.* (2008) Randomized double-blind trial of darbepoetin alfa in patients with symptomatic heart failure and anemia. *Circulation,* **117,** 526–535.

27. Wu, W.C., Rathore, S.S., Wang, Y. *et al.* (2001) Blood transfusion in elderly patients with acute myocardial infarction. *The New England Journal of Medicine,* **345,** 1230–1236.

28. Smith, G.L., Lichtman, J.H., Bracken, M.B. *et al.* (2006) Renal impairment and outcomes in heart failure: systematic review and meta-analysis. *Journal of the American College of Cardiology,* **47,** 1987–1996.

29. Swedberg, K., Kjekshus, J. and Snapinn, S. (1999) Long-term survival in severe heart failure in patients treated with enalapril. Ten year follow-up of CONSENSUS I. *European Heart Journal,* **20,** 136–139.

30. Cohn, J.N., Johnson, G., Ziesche, S. *et al.* (1991) A comparison of enalapril with hydralazine-isosorbide dinitrate in the treatment of chronic congestive heart failure. *The New England Journal of Medicine,* **325,** 303–310.

31. Shlipak, M.G. (2003) Pharmacotherapy for heart failure in patients with renal insufficiency. *Annals of Internal Medicine,* **138,** 917–924.

32. Erdmann, E., Lechat, P., Verkenne, P. *et al.* (2001) Results from post-hoc analyses of the CIBIS II trial: effect of bisoprolol in high-risk patient groups with chronic heart failure. *European Journal of Heart Failure,* **3,** 469–479.

33. Pitt, B., Zannad, F., Remme, W.J. *et al.* for the Randomized Aldactone Evaluation Study Investigators (1999) The effect of spironolactone on morbidity and mortality in patients with severe heart failure. *The New England Journal of Medicine,* **341,** 709–717.

34. Obialo, C.I., Ofili, E.O. and Mirza, T. (2002) Hyperkalemia in congestive heart failure patients aged 63 to 85 years with subclinical renal disease. *The American Journal of Cardiology,* **90,** 663–665.

35. The Digitalis Investigation Group (1997) The effect of digoxin on mortality and morbidity in patients with heart failure. *The New England Journal of Medicine,* **336,** 525–533.

36. Bertoni, A.G., Hundley, W.G., Massing, M.W. *et al.* (2004) Heart failure prevalence, incidence, and mortality in the elderly with diabetes. *Diabetes Care,* **27,** 699–703.

37. Carr, A.A., Kowey, P.R., Devereux, R.B. *et al.* (2005) Hospitalizations for new heart failure among subjects with diabetes mellitus in the RENAAL and LIFE studies. *The American Journal of Cardiology,* **96,** 1530–1536.

38. Stratton, I.M., Adler, A.I., Neil, H.A. *et al.* (2000) Association of glycaemia with macrovascular and microvascular complications of type 2 diabetes (UKPDS 35): prospective observational study. *British Medical Journal,* **321,** 405–412.

39. Eurich, D.T., McAlister, F.A., Blackburn, D.F. *et al.* (2007) Benefits and harms of antidiabetic agents in patients with diabetes and heart failure: systematic review. *British Medical Journal,* **335,** 497–506.

40. Tahrani, A.A., Varughese, G.I., Scarpello, J.H. and Hanna, F.W. (2007) Metformin, heart failure, and lactic acidosis: is metformin absolutely contraindicated? *British Medical Journal,* **335,** 508–512.

41. Masoudi, F.A., Inzucchi, S.E., Wang, Y. *et al.* (2005) Thiazolidinediones, metformin, and outcomes in older patients with diabetes and heart failure: an observational study. *Circulation*, **111**, 583–590.

42. Lago, R.M., Singh, P.P. and Nesto, R.W. (2007) Congestive heart failure and cardiovascular death in patients with prediabetes and type 2 diabetes given thiazolidinediones: a meta-analysis of randomised clinical trials. *Lancet*, **370**, 1129–1136.

43. Le Jemtel, T.H., Padeletti, M. and Jelic, S. (2007) Diagnostic and therapeutic challenges in patients with coexistent chronic obstructive pulmonary disease and chronic heart failure. *Journal of the American College of Cardiology*, **49**, 171–180.

44. Gan, W.Q., Man, S.F., Senthilselvan, A. and Sin, D.D. (2004) Association between chronic obstructive pulmonary disease and systemic inflammation – a systematic review and meta-analysis. *Thorax*, **59**, 574–580.

45. Sidney, S., Sorel, M., Quesenberry, C.P. *et al.* (2005) COPD and incident cardiovascular disease hospitalizations and mortality: Kaiser Permanente Medical Care Program. *Chest*, **128**, 2068–2075.

46. Packard, K., Wurdeman, R. and Arouni, A. (2002) ACE-inhibitor-induced bronchial reactivity in patients with respiratory dysfunction. *Annals of Pharmacotherapy*, **36**, 1058–1067.

47. McAvay, G.J., Van Ness, P.H., Bogardus, S.T. Jr *et al.* (2006) Older adults discharged from the hospital with delirium: 1-year outcomes. *Journal of the American Geriatrics Society*, **54**, 1245–1250.

48. Qiu, C., Winblad, B., Marengoni, A. *et al.* (2006) Heart failure and risk of dementia and Alzheimer disease. *Archives of Internal Medicine*, **166**, 1003–1008.

49. Zuccala, G., Onder, G., Pedone, C. *et al.* (2001) Hypotension and cognitive impairment: selective association in patients with heart failure. *Neurology*, **57**, 1986–1992.

50. Kaduszkiewicz, H., Zimmermann, T., Beck-Bornholdt, H.P. and van den Bussche, H. (2005) Cholinesterase inhibitors for patients with Alzheimer's disease: systematic review of randomised clinical trials. *British Medical Journal*, **331**, 321–327.

51. Inouye, S.K., van Dyck, C.H., Alessi, C.A. *et al.* (1990) Clarifying confusion: The Confusion Assessment Method, a new method for detection of delirium. *Annals of Internal Medicine*, **113**, 941–948.

52. Rutledge, T., Reis, V.A., Linke, S.E. *et al.* (2006) Depression in heart failure: a meta-analytic review of prevalence, intervention effects, and associations with clinical outcomes. *Journal of the American College of Cardiology*, **48**, 1527–1537.

53. Brown, A.M. and Cleland, J.G. (1998) Influence of concomitant disease on patterns of hospitalization in patients with heart failure discharged from Scottish hospitals in 1995. *European Heart Journal*, **19**, 1063–1069.

54. Lip, G.Y.H. and Chung, I. (2006) Antithrombotic therapy for congestive heart failure. *International Journal of Clinical Practice*, **60**, 36–47.

55. Masud, T. and Morris, R. (2001) The epidemiology of falls. *Age and Ageing*, **30** (Suppl 4), S4–S7.

56. Oliver, D., McMurdo, M.E.T. and Patel, S. (2005) Secondary prevention of falls and osteoporotic fractures in older people. *British Medical Journal*, **331**, 123–124.

57. Lawlor, D.A., Patel, R. and Ebrahim, S. (2003) Association between falls in elderly women and chronic diseases and drug use: cross sectional study. *British Medical Journal*, **327**, 712–717.

58. Chang, J.T., Morton, S.C., Rubenstein, L.Z. *et al.* (2004) Interventions for the prevention of falls in older adults: systematic review and meta-analysis of randomised clinical trials. *British Medical Journal*, **328**, 680–683.

59. Bischoff-Ferrari, H.A., Dawson-Hughes, B., Willett, W.C. *et al.* (2004) Effect of vitamin D on falls: a meta-analysis. *The Journal of the American Medical Association*, **291**, 1999–2006.

60. van der Velde, N., Stricker, B.H.C., Pols, H.A.P. and van der Cammen, T.J.M. (2007) Risk of falls after withdrawal of fall-risk-increasing drugs: a prospective cohort study. *British Journal of Clinical Pharmacology*, **63**, 232–237.

61. Podsiadlo, D. and Richardson, S. (1991) The timed "Up & Go": a test of basic functional mobility for frail elderly persons. *Journal of the American Geriatrics Society*, **39**, 142–148.

62. Potocka-Plazak, K. and Plazak, W. (2001) Orthostatic hypotension in elderly women with congestive heart failure. *Aging (Milano)*, **13**, 378–384.

63. Nicola, P.J., Crowson, C.S., Maradit-Kremers, H. *et al.* (2006) Contribution of congestive heart failure and ischemic heart disease to excess mortality in rheumatoid arthritis. *Arthritis and Rheumatism*, **54**, 60–67.

64. Walsh, J.T., Andrews, R., Starling, R. *et al.* (1995) Effects of captopril and oxygen on sleep apnoea in patients with mild to moderate congestive cardiac failure. *British Heart Journal*, **73**, 237–241.

65. Cormican, L.J. and Williams, A. (2005) Sleep disordered breathing and its treatment in congestive heart failure. *Heart*, **91**, 1265–1270.

66. Bradley, T.D., Logan, A.G., Kimoff, R.J. *et al.* (2005) Continuous positive airway pressure for central sleep apnea and heart failure. *The New England Journal of Medicine*, **353**, 2025–2033.

67. Sarkisian, C.A. and Lachs, M.S. (1996) "Failure to thrive" in older adults. *Annals of Internal Medicine*, **124**, 1072–1078.

68. Fried, L.P., Tangen, C.M., Walston, J. *et al.* (2001) Frailty in older adults: evidence for a phenotype. *The Journals of Gerontology. Series A, Biological Sciences, and Medical Sciences*, **56**, M146–M156.

69. Jeter, K.F. and Wagner, D.B. (1990) Incontinence in the American home: a survey of 36,500 people. *Journal of the American Geriatrics Society*, **38**, 379–383.

70. van der Wal, M., Jaarsma, T. and van Veldhuisen, D. (2005) Non-compliance in patients with heart failure: how can we manage it? *European Journal of Heart Failure*, **7**, 5–17.

71. Kenny, A.M., Boxer, R., Walsh, S. *et al.* (2006) Femoral bone mineral density in patients with heart failure. *Osteoporosis International*, **17**, 1420–1427.

72. Rossouw, J.E., Anderson, G.L., Prentice, R.L. *et al.* (2002) Risks and benefits of estrogen plus progestin in healthy postmenopausal women: principal results from the Women's Health Initiative randomized controlled trial. *The Journal of the American Medical Association*, **288**, 321–333.

73. Lim, L.S., Fink, H.A. and Kuskowski, M.A. (2008) Loop diuretic use and increased rates of hip bone loss in older men: the osteoporotic fractures in men study. *Archives of Internal Medicine*, **168**, 735–740.

74. Schoofs, M.W., van der Klift, M., Hofman, A. *et al.* (2003) Thiazide diuretics and the risk for hip fracture. *Annals of Internal Medicine*, **139**, 476–482.

9

Treatment and management in primary care

Alan Begg

University of Dundee Townhead Practice, Links Health Centre, Montrose

---

Key messages

- Patients with suspected heart failure should have ECG ± BNP estimation (if available) at the time of their initial consultation, in order to promptly identify those who require echocardiography to confirm the diagnosis.

- The ability of older patients to comply with complex drug regimens should be assessed and, if required, measures introduced to improve compliance and reduce side effects.

- Adherence to local treatment guidelines is important to ensure that medication and other therapies are optimized.

- All patients should be reviewed at least every 6 months based on local management protocols.

- All general practices in the UK are required to maintain accurate and regularly updated patient data files, with copies of hospital correspondence for all coronary heart disease patients, including those with heart failure.

A Practical Guide to Heart Failure in Older People, Edited by C Ward and M D Witham
© 2009 John Wiley & Sons, Ltd

9.1   Introduction

Collaboration between primary and secondary care, and coordination of the service provided across these two sectors, is essential for the good management of patients with heart failure of all ages. This is especially so for older patients with advanced heart failure, whose disease course is typified by recurrent episodes of hospitalization and/or frequent visits to a heart failure clinic or from a heart failure nurse.

Patients with heart failure live either at home, in sheltered accommodation, a care home or a nursing home. It is therefore important that those working in secondary care have an understanding of the primary care management structure, the processes for data collection, as well as documentation and audit. It is also important to be aware of what is achievable within this structure, and an appreciation of the problems of treating a growing population of older patients with complex medical and social needs. Without this understanding, coordination of effective care will inevitably suffer.

9.2   The role of primary care and the patient population

Patient profile and workload

General practice has a key role in the diagnosis, investigation and management of all patients with heart failure (HF). The majority of these patients are managed throughout the course of their disease by their general practitioners, with most of their care taking place in the community. The average age of a heart failure patient seen in general practice is 75 years for men, and 79 for women [1]. Many of the women will have a long history of hypertension and are likely to have preserved left ventricular (LV) systolic function (see Chapter 2). Cardiologists, in contrast, are more likely to see younger male patients with an average age of 64, who will have LV systolic dysfunction often resulting from a previous myocardial infarction [2].

A patient with heart failure consults their general practitioner (GP) on average between three and 11 times each year [3,4]. This workload is likely to increase overall with the increasing prevalence of heart failure due to the ageing of the population, and with more patients surviving a coronary event but subsequently succumbing to heart failure. Patients usually present first of all to their GP when symptoms become apparent. The initial assessment of their history and clinical signs will determine what investigations, if any, are arranged to establish a diagnosis, and which medication is commenced. It will also determine the ongoing care and monitoring that is likely to be put in place.

A GP in the UK, and other members of the primary care team, have a contractual obligation under the quality and outcomes framework to ensure that patients with suspected heart failure have the diagnosis confirmed, are added to a properly maintained register, and that follow-up care is arranged. This care needs to be coordinated with other professionals such as specialist heart failure nurses who may be involved in the patient's care, as well as other members of the secondary care team. Although the basic quality standards to which the GP should adhere are at present agreed nationally, the process of caring varies significantly from practice to practice, depending not only on the practice arrangements but also on local circumstances. These different circumstances and arrangements may affect the overall quality of care and lead to difficulties in following guideline-driven evidence-based practice. These factors include:

- The resources and level of care available in the primary care organization
- Local facilities and the specific arrangements which are in place
- The availability of echocardiography and BNP testing
- The provision of a specialist heart failure nurse service.

9.3 Heart failure registers, data collection and audit

Heart failure registers

The National Service Framework (NSF) for Coronary Heart Disease (CHD) [5] set the milestone that, by April 2001, every primary care team should systematically develop and maintain a practice-based CHD register which was to include people with HF. In addition, all medical records and hospital correspondence was to be held in date order so that data could be readily retrieved. Drug therapy lists were to be created for all patients on long-term therapy. This register of patients was to be the basis for providing active structured follow-up care for people with HF based on locally agreed protocols (Table 9.1).

The use of accurate disease registers forms the basis of the modern approach to the management of long-term conditions in the UK and other western societies. Disease registers provide a direct means of identifying patients with a specific diagnosis, allowing them to be called and recalled for monitoring. Once the necessary information which is felt to be the most appropriate for collection is added to the disease register, all aspects of the patient's care can be audited.

For a patient presenting to their GP with suspected HF, a sequence of specific actions is necessary for effective ongoing care. A diagnosis needs to be accurately confirmed, and then given an appropriate clinical code so that it can be included in the appropriate register [6]. This allows the patients to be easily identified, their

Table 9.1 Components of locally agreed practice protocols for managing people with suspected heart failure.

Appropriate patient assessment – including risk factors, symptoms and signs
Relevant investigations – including ECG, echocardiography and biochemistry
Referral arrangements for echocardiography – investigation should be carried out by a trained
   operator to an agreed competency standard
Lifestyle advice
Appropriate therapy
Indications for referral
Provision of patient education and family support
Arrangements for follow-up and review
Communication standards required between all health professionals
Annual audit of care of heart failure patients

details retrieved and ongoing monitoring simplified; structured care and clinical audit can then take place.

The publication of the NSF was the first step in this structured process, and set the basis and stimulus for the creation of HF registers within general practice.

Quality and outcomes framework (QOF) General Practice

The QOF was introduced into United Kingdom general practice in April 2004. It consists of 10 different disease categories made up of clinical indicators relevant to the individual disease category. Points are awarded for undertaking tasks such as creating a disease register, or for reaching a certain level of achievement, which is then reflected in the doctors' remuneration. The indicators are set to define clear standards of care which can be easily measured, ideally from an electronic clinical database. These indicators were developed mainly from recommendations within national clinical guidelines especially those derived from high levels of clinical evidence.

The initial stage of the QOF included a subsection of the CHD category covering left ventricular systolic dysfunction (LVSD) in patients with CHD. This initial group was chosen because systolic dysfunction secondary to underlying CHD was regarded as the most common cause of HF in general practice patients. Patients with HF associated with preserved systolic function (HF-PSF) were clearly stated to be outside the scope of the clinical indicators being measured at this time.

The clinical indicators were updated in 2006 [7] as these narrow inclusion criteria were felt to exclude as many as 50% of patients with HF [8]. It was also noted that, of all the cardiovascular diseases, it was the prevalence of HF that was increasing the most, and that it was associated with a poor quality of life and prognosis and with major financial implications.

Data coding

READ codes are currently the standard coding system used nationally across the UK in general practice for computer recording of clinical information. This system can be used to record individual signs, symptoms and diagnosis on a hierarchically arranged basis. Procedures, processes and investigations can also be individually coded which allows the clinician easy access to data concerning the patient's management. In the case of a patient with HF, the whole process of care can be individually coded (Table 9.2). This can include, in addition to main symptoms and signs, whether or not an ECG or echocardiogram has been ordered and performed, its result, and whether specialist referral has been made. This is in addition to recording all medications prescribed and dates for recall and follow-up.

The use of this clinical coding system allows standardization of data indexing and storage which can then be easily retrieved and aggregated. This standardization also reduces variation in data collection which in turn helps to improve clinical care and aids audit and research.

Table 9.2 READ Codes used to identify patients with heart failure.

G58.00	Heart failure
G58.11	Cardiac failure
G580.00	Congestive heart failure
G580.11	Congestive cardiac failure
G580.12	Right heart failure
G580.13	Right ventricular failure
G580.14	Biventricular failure
G580000	Acute congestive heart failure
G580100	Chronic congestive heart failure
G580200	Decompensated cardiac failure
G580300	Compensated cardiac failure
G581.00	Left ventricular failure
G581.11	Asthma – cardiac
G581.12	Pulmonary oedema – acute
G581.13	Impair left ventricular function
G581000	Acute left ventricular failure
G582.00	Acute heart failure
G58200	Heart failure NOS[a]
G582.11	Weak heart
G582.12	Cardiac failure NOS[a]
G1yz100	Rheumatic left ventricular failure
662G.00	New York Heart Association classification Class I
662g.00	New York Heart Association classification Class II
662h.00	New York Heart Association classification Class III
662i.00	New York Heart Association classification Class IV

[a]NOS Not Specified.

SNOMED CT (Systematized Nomenclature of Medicine - Clinical Terms) was created in early 2002 by the merger of the original College of American Pathologies SNOMED system with READ codes, but this differs from the ICD (International Classification of Diseases) codes used for hospital discharge data which are used to analyze morbidity and mortality data from a variety of sources. Currently, both systems operate in parallel, although individual codes can be mapped across the two systems to allow comparisons to be made. In order to remain accurate, this requires definitions to be similar, although in an ideal world one system would be used for recording both the diagnosis and the process of care.

Clinical indicators for heart failure in general practice

The indicators in use from 2004 to 2006 (Table 9.3) applied only to patients with a diagnosis of LVSD secondary to underlying CHD. The diagnosis of LVSD was to be based on the result of an echocardiogram, which was seen as the most important single investigation in patients with HF. The guidance accepted that an echocardiogram may not be possible in all patients, with those who were frail and immobile specifically mentioned. The diagnosis was to be prospective and only applied to those diagnosed after a given date, on the basis that the provision of an echocardiography service had not been universal in the past and that the diagnosis of HF had probably been made mainly on clinical grounds. This encouraged practices to re-examine diagnoses made previously and, with the passage of time, registers would be much more accurate. There was however provision to exclude patients from the need to establish an accurate diagnosis so as not to penalize remuneration where it was logistically impossible to have an echocardiogram. Primary care organizations were encouraged to commission such a service as a priority, and this resulted in a significant increase in provision in recent years across the UK. Once diagnosed, these patients were expected to be treated with an ACE inhibitor or an angiotensin 2 receptor antagonist. These tentative first steps, although limited in who was included and in their scope, did help to encourage the development of heart failure services. They also provided a platform for further expansion to include all patients with LVSD or heart failure with preserved systolic function (HF-PSF), no matter what the underlying aetiology. From 2006 onwards (Table 9.3), all patients with HF were to be included on the register, irrespective of the aetiology – that is, not only those with LVSD due to CHD but those with HF-PSF. In addition to the diagnosis being confirmed by echocardiography, confirmation by specialist assessment was also accepted. This specialist could be a GP with a specialist clinical interest in HF, but it also allowed for the inclusion of patients in whom the diagnosis had been confirmed by cardiac scintigraphy or angiography. The requirement to treat with an ACE inhibitor or an angiotensin 2 receptor antagonist still applied, in line with the evidence, but only to those patients where the HF had been confirmed as being due to

Table 9.3 General practice clinical indicators.

	2004 Left ventricular failure	Points		2006 Heart failure	Points
LVD1	Practices should produce a register of patients with CHD and LVD	4	HF1	The practice can produce a register of patients with heart failure	4
LVD2	Percentage of patients with CHD and LVD who have had a diagnosis made after 1st April 2003 confirmed by echocardiogram	6	HF2	Percentage of patients with a diagnosis of heart failure made after 1st April 2006 confirmed by echocardiogram or by specialist assessment	6
	Percentage of patients with a diagnosis of CHD and LVD who are currently treated with an ACE inhibitor or angiotensin-receptor blocker	10	HF3	Percentage of patients with a diagnosis of heart failure due to LVD currently treated with an ACE inhibitor or angiotensin-receptor blocker who can tolerate therapy with no contraindication	10
			HF4[a]	Percentage of patients with a diagnosis of heart failure due to LVD who are currently treated with an ACE inhibitor or angiotensin-receptor blocker treated with a beta-blocker licensed for heart failure	9

[a]QOF Changes and New Indicators for 2009/10
http://www.bma.org.uk/ap.nsf/AttachmentsByTitle/PDFQOFchanges200910/$FILE/QOFchanges200910.pdf.

Table 9.4   READ codes used to identify patients with current diagnosis of heart failure due to left ventricular dysfunction.

G581	Left ventricular failure
585f.00	Echocardiogram shows left ventricular systolic dysfunction
585g.00	Echocardiogram shows left ventricular diastolic dysfunction
G5yyA00	Left ventricular systolic dysfunction
G5yyA00	Left ventricular diastolic dysfunction

LVSD. This meant that patients with LVSD had to be identified for monitoring and verification purposes as a subsection of the heart failure register (Table 9.4). The addition of treatment with a beta-blocker as a clinical indicator, although desirable (and making clinical sense), will be included in the foreseeable future despite the competing demands to include new disease categories and organisational aspects into the new QOF (Table 9.3).

9.4   Heart failure in general practice

Epidemiology in primary care

Among a population study consisting of a cross-sectional group of 1640 men and women aged between 25 and 74 years who were screened for LVSD, 1.5% had symptomatic and 1.4% asymptomatic LVSD, defined as a left ventricular ejection fraction (LVEF) $\leq$30%. The prevalence differed significantly between men and women (4% versus 2%), and increased with age in both genders. In the 65–74-year age group the rates were 6.4% for men (3.2% symptomatic) and 4.9% for women (3.6% symptomatic) [9].

In the Heart of England Study, 3960 randomly selected patients from general practice underwent a full screening process for LVSD and heart failure. Among these patients, 1.86% had definite LVSD, but the figure rose to 3.6% in those aged over 75 years. Based on the data from this study the minimum prevalence for definite heart failure was given as 2.3% [8]. The prevalence of 3.7% in patients aged 70–84 years compared with a rate of 7.5% determined in a study carried out in general practice in southern England [10].

The prevalence of LVSD in 500 older patients selected from a cohort of 5002 patients aged $\geq$70 years living at home in a Welsh practice was rather higher, at 9.8% [11]. A retrospective review of the medical records [12] of patients registered with two Liverpool practices indicated that 60% of the females diagnosed with heart failure were aged 75 or over, the equivalent figure in males being 38%. Continuous morbidity recording from 71 general practices in Scotland in 1999 identified heart failure as the second most common reason for consultation in males and females aged 85 and over. Among males aged 75–84, heart failure was the fourth most common reason given for consultation, although it did not feature in the top five reasons in those aged 74 or under.

The QOF data should provide a more current and accurate indication of the prevalence of heart failure in UK practices. Prevalence is seen as a measure of the level of a condition at a specified time, and is collected from each practice on National Prevalence Day, currently the last day in March each year; a national prevalence figure is published soon afterwards.

Unadjusted practice figures are the percentage of patients on the register compared to the number of patients registered with the practice, and provide an indication of a national prevalence rate when figures from all practices are collated at a national level. They take no account of age, gender or other differences between practices, and may possibly be affected by the availability of a specific local service, local diagnostic practice, as well as how complete and accurate the practice records are.

The estimated national prevalence rate for heart failure in England for 2007/08 was given as 0.75 per 100 patients registered to GPS. The equivalent figure for Wales was 0.95, for Northern Ireland 0.8, and for Scotland 0.86, with the UK average being 0.84 at present [13]. This is based on figures given in the register for heart failure, which includes all patients with a diagnosis of heart failure, the corresponding value for LV dysfunction in England being 0.38 in 2007/08, 0.38 in Northern Ireland, and 0.5 in Wales, with the Scottish value for 2007/08 being 0.62. A direct comparison of the LVSD figure with previous years is difficult, as the register for LV dysfunction prior to 2006 applied only to patients with this diagnosis and who also had confirmed CHD. The current LVSD average for the whole of the UK is given as 0.47.

Currently, we are beginning to see a degree of consistency in the published QOF figures for prevalence across the UK and this may reflect to a certain extent the uniformity and standardization in confirming the diagnosis. This contrasts with the variation seen in population- and practice-based studies which use a variety of differing diagnostic criteria.

Workload

The continuous morbidity recording in Scottish general practices [4] provides an overview of the likely workload for general practice resulting from patients with heart failure (Table 9.5). This information was recorded onto the GPASS (General Practice Administration System for Scotland) computer system for each face-to-face contact between a GP and a patient. These contacts included surgery consultations and home visits; out-of-hours contacts were recorded when GPs were responsible for all care in the community, with the data collated centrally.

Table 9.5   Scottish general practitioners' consultations for heart failure.

Rates per 1000 practice population

40 general practices in 1998

	Consultation rate	Incidence rate	Prevalence rate
	Based on number of consultations at which diagnosis is recorded	Based on first or recurrence diagnoses recorded during time period	Based on no patients with at least first recurrence or persistent diagnosis
Male			
All ages	16.4	4.2	6.6
65–74	68.7	17.3	25.9
75–84	159.3	40.2	65.6
85 and over	262.9	69.0	100.8
Female			
All ages	18	5.6	7.9
65–74	58.9	19	25.2
75–84	128.3	36.8	53.3
85 and over	184.4	47.6	78.9

Presenting symptoms and baseline investigations

The presenting symptoms which make a GP suspect the possibility of cardiac failure have such a low specificity that the diagnosis may be far from clear at the outset. This low specificity of heart failure symptoms may decrease further with increasing age. The GP should, however, have access to a full past medical history which may well include conditions that are either causes or risk factors for heart failure. Similarly, the list of previous medical diagnoses may include conditions that need to be considered in the differential diagnosis based on the presenting symptoms (Table 9.6). A clinical examination may provide further pointers towards the actual diagnosis, but both the variability of the presence of specific signs, as well as the skills of the GP, may be a limiting factor. Nonetheless, the presence of a severe symptom in a patient who is clearly unwell, with the presence of signs such as a tachyarrhythmia, heart murmur or basal crepitations, may necessitate hospital admission. Once admitted to a medical receiving unit, investigation and initiation of treatment can be instigated much more easily.

For patients who are to be managed in the community, basic investigations as well as objective tests need to be undertaken in order to confirm or exclude the diagnosis (Tables 9.7 and 9.8). Local circumstances will determine whether BNP

Table 9.6 Characteristics of patients suspected of having heart failure by their general practitioner ($n = 458$).

Males (%)	40.2
Mean age (years)	72.6
Symptoms (%)	
Dyspnoea	87.3
Oedema	65.9
Tiredness	55.5
Orthopnoea	46.0
Paroxysmal nocturnal dyspnoea	61.0
Wheeze	17.6
Cough	20.3
Past medical history (%)	
Angina	38.4
Myocardial infarction	19.4
Coronary revascularization	7.6
Hypertension	47.6

Adapted from Ref. [16].

Table 9.7 General Practitioner initial investigations of patients with heart failure.

Bloods	Full blood count
	Urea and electrolytes
	Thyroid-stimulating hormone
	Liver function tests
	Glucose level
	Lipid profile
	BNP (B-type natriuretic peptide)
Urinalysis	Check for presence of protein and glucose
12-lead electrocardiogram	
Chest X-ray	
Echocardiogram	

Table 9.8 Key requirements for GPs to effectively manage patients with heart failure.

BNP testing	Provision of local service
ECG	Provision of service and training in interpretation
Echocardiogram	Open or easy access with clear explanation of results
Titration of medication	Assistance of specialist heart failure nurse
Specialist help	Access to advice or clinic for complicated cases

measurement, ECG or echocardiogram can be carried out to either confirm or exclude the diagnosis. Determining the cause is also imperative to allow the patient to be properly managed on the basis of current guidance.

Use of the ECG in General Practice

Recording a 12-lead ECG is an important initial step in general practice when investigating a patient with suspected heart failure. Although many practices now have access to an ECG machine, a lack of equipment is still a factor in this test not being performed prior to referral. One study, however, did record that 49% of patients referred with a suspected diagnosis of heart failure had previously had an ECG [14]. In another study of 534 patients aged between 17 and 94 years, all had had an ECG recorded prior to referral for open access echocardiography [15]. This was one of several reports which concluded that LV dysfunction is very unlikely if the electrocardiogram is normal, or shows only minor abnormalities. In a similar study of 458 symptomatic patients suspected by their GP of having heart failure, the sensitivity of the ECG for LVSD and heart failure was 97% and 95%, respectively [16].

Although concerns have been expressed as to whether an ECG is an adequate screening tool in patients with suspected heart failure [17], it remains an important step as a 'rule-out test' to exclude the diagnosis, and should be performed on all patients suspected of having heart failure. General practitioners tend to express a lack of confidence in interpreting ECGs, especially as changes may be subtle, or because they lack the necessary interpretation skills. As a result, specialist input may still be necessary to accurately identify ECG abnormalities [18,19]. One study has shown that pre-echocardiography ECG screening by GPs of patients who had consulted their GP with symptoms suggestive of heart failure for LVSD had a mean sensitivity of 0.94 (95% CI = 0.92–0.95) and a mean specificity of 0.58 (95% CI = 0.56–0.60) [20]. However, when compared to hospital practitioners, the interpretation by GPs had a significantly lower sensitivity and a poorer negative predictive value. In this particular study, the sensitivity and specificity was 53% and 63% respectively, compared to 95% and 47% [21].

The increased use of an interpretive ECG recording machine has the potential to increase the confidence of those in primary care in their interpretation of ECGs. A Danish study [22] showed that GPs were good at correcting false positive diagnoses made by an interpretive ECG recording. It remains the general rule, however, that interpretation should not be accepted without consideration of the clinical context and a visual inspection of the ECG trace.

Use of BNP in Primary Care

The measurement of B-type natriuretic peptide (BNP), either in the laboratory or as a point-of-care test, has the potential to provide GPs with an additional tool in deciding whether a patient with suspected heart failure should be referred for further assessment; this may be more appropriate for GPs who either do not record ECGs in their own practice or who are not confident in confirming an automated ECG report. A normal BNP test can be used to effectively rule out a diagnosis of heart failure, with the ECG providing additional information in these circumstances [23]. The GP is then in a position to consider a noncardiac cause for the patient's symptoms, thus avoiding the need to commence therapy whilst awaiting for the outcome of an echocardiogram.

Echocardiography

A lack of access to echocardiography is seen as a major barrier in the establishment of a diagnosis of heart failure in primary care [24] yet it is acknowledged as being essential to confirm the diagnosis and to guide management [19]. General practitioners report that open-access echocardiography is not always used, even when available. This may be in part due to patient choice, especially in those patients who are ill, infirm or unwilling to attend an outpatient appointment. There is also a perception that reports tend to be too technical and that GPs are unable to understand the information given without the addition of a clinical opinion on the echocardiogram interpretation [18]. An echocardiogram provides information on the structure and function of the chambers of the heart, the valves and the pericardium, but referring all patients with possible heart failure has in the past had significant service implications. However, an improved access to this investigation provides a more comprehensive clarification on the presence or absence of LVSD in patients with suspected heart failure. Although an echocardiogram service can be established in general practice premises [25], it is important that the establishment of any service should ensure equity of access and takes local geographical and service provision factors into account. It should also make full use of the presence of local expertise such as GPs with a specialist interest who can operate such a service.

Open-access echocardiography is defined as a request for investigation by a GP, without prior assessment by a cardiologist [26]. The demand for such a service has been driven by the publication of the National Service Framework for CHD and the QOF which highlight the need to confirm or exclude a definitive diagnosis.

The benefits of an open-access referral system are earlier diagnosis and treatment, with a reduction in both waiting times and also the possible burden on secondary care. Three of the studies included in a systematic review of open-access echocardiography reported normal findings in 46%, 54% and 74% of the patients referred, with the mean percentage of impaired systolic function in four of the studies being 19%. The majority of primary care referrals for open-access echocardiography were for suspected heart failure, but in one study only 12% of referrals were considered to be inappropriate [27]. This review did conclude, however, that there was a lack of rigorously controlled studies to support the widespread establishment of an open-access echocardiography service [26]. It is nevertheless important that when an open-access service is established, appropriate educational material and information is provided to guide the GP in their clinical management, based on the result of the echocardiogram.

9.5   Treatment and management

Guideline-based treatment

Current guidelines on the diagnosis and management of heart failure may not be familiar to many GPs, who feel uncertain as to which of the many available guidelines they should follow. However, national evidence-based guidelines have informed the National Service Framework for CHD and the QOF, which have in turn led to a change in clinical practice. There are now numerous local guidelines based on the principles of practice and treatment published in national and international guidelines, but adapted to reflect the availability of service provision locally. It is important, however, when drawing up these local guidelines not to deviate from the evidence underpinning the guideline recommendations; differing local circumstances on how care is delivered may make a difference to outcomes, including the availability of echocardiogram services, BNP testing and a defined heart failure service. Primary care requires local protocols which are relevant to the local situation.

Deviation from guideline-based treatment

There has been a tendency in the past, that when a patient presented with symptoms and signs suggestive of heart failure, to treat them with a diuretic and to monitor their individual response. Depending on such response (and an improvement is common as diuretics will, for some time, reduce congestive symptoms), the patient might continue on this medication in the long term. Ideally, however, they should also be referred for further assessment or for investigation to confirm the diagnosis. The less-aggressive approach has tended to be used more in older people, especially in those with multiple comorbidities. However, this can lead to patients being denied effective evidence-based treatment such as ACE inhibitors or beta-blockers. The GPs' concerns are at least partly responsible for this situation, notably relating to the introduction and titration of these medications, a fear of poly-pharmacy, and worries about undesirable side effects such as hypotension and subsequent impaired renal function. These concerns remain, and so this approach may continue, although in order to ensure the quality of care and to comply with the demands of the QOF, there is currently less leeway to deviate from an evidence-based approach. The wishes and general condition of the patient however must be considered with a management plan, personal requirements and care provision developed around individual needs.

Referral for specialist advice

The reasons why a GP might refer a patient for specialist opinion, assessment or for inpatient care are complex and varied (Table 9.9). They depend on the expertise of the doctor and on locally available procedures and facilities, as well as the needs of the

Table 9.9 Indications for referral for specialist advice.

Category	
Investigation	To confirm a diagnosis To determine underlying cause
Pharmacotherapy	For decision on initiation of therapy Advice on complex pharmacotherapy
Laboratory[a]	Deteriorating renal function, Serum creatinine $>150\,\mu mol\,l^{-1}$ Hyponatraemia $<135\,mmol\,l^{-1}$ (ESC)[a] Hyperkalaemia $\geq 6\,mmol\,l^{-1}$ (ESC)[a] Anaemia
Physical	Symptoms not controlled or not responding to treatment Step change in condition or patient unstable with severe heart failure Symptomatic hypotension or asymptomatic hypotension with SBP $<90\,mmHg$ (SIGN 95) Pathological weight gain
Cardiology	Significant murmur or confirmed valvular disease Atrial fibrillation Symptomatic arrhythmia
Care of the elderly	Diagnostic uncertainty Multiple inter-related comorbidities
Social	Home management becoming less effective Difficulty in providing care at home

Recommendations from other guidelines:
[a]European Society of Cardiology [28]: Specialist advice should be sought if: 1. Serum sodium $<135\,mmol\,l^{-1}$; 2. Serum creatinine $>150\,mmol\,l^{-1}$; 3. Serum potassium $<6.0\,mmol\,l^{-1}$ 'is acceptable'.
American Heart Association/American College of Cardiology [29]: 1. Serum creatinine $>221\,mmol\,l^{-1}$; 2. Serum potassium $>5.5\,mmol\,l^{-1}$.

patient. Referral may be to a cardiology or care of the elderly clinic, or there may be a dedicated heart failure outpatient service or rapid access clinic. In certain areas GPs with a special interest in heart failure are increasingly seen as the key to service provision, providing a local clinic service for their colleagues across a primary care area. This service however can only be provided in conjunction with secondary care and other components of a heart failure service. Good communication between all practitioners involved is essential to ensure continuity of care and comprehensive service provision.

For these reasons, it is difficult to provide a definitive list of which patients should be referred by primary care for more specialized assessment and ongoing care. Some of the categories that should be considered are outlined in Table 9.9.

Structured care in the community

Once patients are stable there is a need for regular review to be carried out in primary care. For patients with CHD the QOF stipulates that this review should be carried out within given time intervals which, for patients with CHD, should be on an annual basis. Multidisciplinary disease management programmes for patients with CHD have been shown to have a beneficial effect on the uptake of secondary prevention drugs and addressing risk factors [30]. It seems appropriate that patients with heart failure should be included in this process with a regular review interval of six months not being unreasonable, considering the potential for deterioration and other complications. Routine reviews should be carried out in a structured manner, while the use of an agreed template will ensure that all aspects of care are covered by this review process.

Components of this review should include:

- Reviewing details of recent hospital admissions

- Addressing new problems

- Assessing current symptoms and mental status

- Performing an appropriate examination

- Recording an ECG may be necessary if there is doubt about the cardiac rhythm

- A full medication review with the computer repeat record being updated

- Arrangements should be made for routine laboratory investigations – to include renal function, electrolytes and a full blood count

- Annual influenza immunization should be given if due and the pneumococcal immunization status should be checked

- The opportunity should be taken to address and reinforce the need for lifestyle change

- Arrangements should be made to address any new or current social issues.

Any specific concerns should be addressed at the time of review, or followed up in liaison with the appropriate member of the multidisciplinary team or the heart failure nurse.

A heart failure service (see also chapter 13)

Although patients with heart failure may initially present to their GP, a dedicated heart failure service is increasingly recognized as pivotal in the care of these patients. A multidisciplinary team approach centres on identifying which member of the team has the most appropriate skills or expertise to deal with each specific aspect of care. Local services and team composition, as well as whether the practice is urban or rural, will have a bearing on how care is delivered. Reduced mobility may make attendance at the GP's surgery, an outpatient clinic, day or general hospital extremely difficult. Many of these patients are elderly with increased physical and social needs and with limited scope for self care, but as far as possible they should be cared for in their own home. In many cases they will be looked after by family or relatives, but often the need for residential or nursing home care will arise. Arrangements will often have to be made for domiciliary visits as clinic attendance may be extremely difficult and exhausting for the patient. The presence of local day care facilities can be beneficial and help to improve the level of care provided, but an appropriate means of transport needs to be considered and provided as required.

Other members of the practice-based team – practice nurses, health care assistants, practice pharmacist and community nurse – will all be involved, and it is essential that there is good communication between these professionals in order to provide coordinated care and avoid any duplication in that care. Care in the community services can often operate at arm's length from the health services, with the patient's personal care being provided by social care officers. Such personnel need to be appropriately trained and to understand their role in monitoring the patient, especially as they will often attend the patient on a daily basis. A lack of continuity of carers can often lead to difficulties, as frequent changes of carers will not help the patient's confidence. Communication within the social care team and with the medical care team must be paramount if effective continuity of care is to be provided.

A Cochrane review on heart failure service organization [31] grouped the interventions into multidisciplinary, case management or clinic attendance. The first approach was felt to possibly reduce heart failure-related admissions in the short term, but the second approach is more likely to lead to reduced all-cause mortality but with weaker evidence for reductions in admissions for heart failure. There was no evidence of benefit for the third approach, and of all the interventions described the involvement of a specialist nurse was common to all the studies reviewed.

A study examining the effect of a disease management programme for patients with chronic heart failure in primary care may inform us on how a peripatetic nurse specialist, travelling between practices to hold regular clinics, may be the answer to coordinated structured care. It may also help address what are seen as some of the current problems with hospital-based heart failure services, which may not allow for rural situations and different ways of working in different practices [32]. This nurse intervention included patient assessment, confirmation of diagnosis by investigation, medication management and titration, home visits for housebound patients and liaison between primary and secondary care. The nurse had the facility to refer patients for echocardiography and also to a secondary care cardiology clinic which had access to additional cardiological investigations. This direct involvement at the primary care level by the specialist nurse taking responsibility for heart failure case management may allow a truly multidisciplinary approach, with all team members playing an appropriate part.

9.6   Specific problems in treating older patients

Medication

Any proposed changes in medication instituted by a heart failure nurse, a hospital clinic or following hospitalization must be communicated to the practice, which should develop a system to ensure that the medication and repeat prescribing record is kept up-to-date at all times.

Older people can be poorly motivated to take their medication, especially if they are aware of its side effects. Other barriers to safe treatment include difficulty in understanding complex dosing regimens, titration and flexible dosing, and identifying specific tablets – such as which one is the diuretic. Visual impairment in older people can also create difficulties at all stages of medication provision. Monitored dosage systems can help with the self-management of medication, but they do not overcome the problem of flexible dosing on a day-to-day basis. Compliance aids such as wing-topped bottles, tailored medication charts, large-print labels and compartmental devices can help. However, although the latter can act as a visual prompt to show that a medication has been taken, fine adaptive skills are often required to remove the tablets from the box.

Communication

Difficulties in communicating with older patients with heart failure may be due to associated confusion, cognitive impairment or deafness. Any explanation of the condition, prognosis, medication and course of action should take this into account, and education programmes should be tailored accordingly with partners, close relatives and carers being involved as far as possible when the information is delivered. Deafness and difficulty communicating by telephone may mean that a telephone monitoring approach may not be an appropriate and reliable means of monitoring the older age group. Problems may also arise in re-ordering medication, and rigid repeat prescription systems may also be inappropriate with flexibility and assistance required.

Lifestyle

Older patients may be reluctant to change their lifestyle and routine unless they are able to appreciate the benefits. Self-management programmes, if used, should take into account potential difficulties such as the risk of falls when attempting to weigh oneself, as well as the possible difficulty of taking an accurate reading. Community meals do not always cater for specific dietary needs or tastes, so other nutritional approaches may need to be considered.

Primary and secondary prevention

Heart failure has a poor prognosis, and a more appropriate strategy than 'waiting for it to happen' is to address aggressively its risk factors with the aim of preventing or delaying its development. At present, there is no comprehensive national strategy for the primary prevention of CHD, the main risk factor for the development of heart failure. It is likely, however, that in the near future – at least in England – a screening programme will be introduced nationally to screen the population for their cardiovascular risk. If steps are then taken to reduce that risk, the subsequent reduction of CHD should lead in time to a reduction of heart failure. A related issue is the need for secondary preventive measures for the increased numbers of patients surviving a coronary event and who are therefore at a particularly high risk of heart failure. The QOF does have incentives for general practice to increase the uptake of such secondary preventive measures, with the aim of reducing future events. In a similar way, targets are set for patients with hypertension and blood pressure-lowering which similarly, with time, should reduce coronary events and left ventricular hypertrophy as another main risk factor for heart failure. Also included in the quality and outcome measures are indicators to reduce the complications of diabetes, chronic kidney disease and atrial fibrillation, as well improving the control of patients with chronic obstructive pulmonary disease (COPD), each of which in different ways contributes to the problems associated with heart failure. Primary care also has a responsibility to encourage the reduction of traditional risk factors such as smoking and alcohol intake.

Another specific and increasing problem is that of obesity. After adjustment for other risk factors, obesity can increase the risk of heart failure by up to 100% [33]. The prevalence of obesity given as a body mass index greater than $30 \, kg \, m^{-2}$ is increasing in the UK population, although at present incentivized activity in primary care is restricted to identifying only those patients who can then be targeted for future interventions. Of the main risk factors for heart failure, only valvular disease is not covered by quality targets. Aortic valve calcification is associated with an inflammatory process and endothelial injury in a similar way to that seen in atherosclerosis, and it shares traditional risk factors such as smoking, hypertension, diabetes and hyperlipidaemia with CHD. Addressing the modifiable risk factors for CHD may reduce the risk of developing calcification. It has also been postulated that statins may stabilize the lesions of cardiac atherosclerotic valves and retard the calcification process [34], although clinical trials conducted to date have provided mixed results [35,36]. Mitral annular calcification, which is seen more in older people and produces the same clinical effect as mitral stenosis or regurgitation, is also associated with hypertension, diabetes and hyperlipidaemia [37]. In a similar way, aggressive risk factor modification in the younger age groups may prevent its development at a later age.

Any significant murmur which is picked up on an opportunistic basis should be fully assessed and investigated, with easy access to echocardiography and specialist cardiology being especially important. Effective early intervention in these cases could reduce the risk of subsequent heart failure.

References

1. de Giuli, F., Khaw, K.T., Cowie, M.R. *et al.* (2005) Incidence and outcome of persons with a clinical diagnosis of heart failure in a general practice population of 696,884 in the United Kingdom. *European Journal of Heart Failure*, **7** (3), 295–302.
2. Mosterd, A. and Hoes, A.W. (2007) Clinical epidemiology of heart failure. *Heart*, **93** (9), 1137–1146.
3. Patel, K.C.R., Prince, J., Mirza, S. and Edmonds, L. (2008) Evaluation of an open-access heart failure service spanning primary and secondary care. *British Journal of Cardiology*, **15**, 35–39.
4. GP consultations, incidence and prevalence rates. (1999) Information Services Division Scotland. Available at http://www.isdscotland.org/isd/401.html.
5. Department of Health (2000) Coronary heart disease: national service framework for coronary heart disease – modern standards and service models. Available at http://www.dh.gov.uk/en/Publicationsandstatistics/Publications/PublicationsPolicyAndGuidance/DH_4094275.

6. General Practitioners Committee (2003) *New GMS Contract. Investing in General Practice*. The NHS Federation, British Medical Association, London.

7. NHS Employers (2006/07) *Revisions to the GMS Contract. Delivering Investment in General Practice*. British Medical Association, London.

8. Davies, M., Hobbs, F., Davis, R. *et al.* (2001) Prevalence of left-ventricular systolic dysfunction and heart failure in the Echocardiographic Heart of England Screening study: a population based study. *Lancet*, **358**, 439–444.

9. McDonagh, T.A., Morrison, C.E., Lawrence, A. *et al.* (1997) Symptomatic and asymptomatic left-ventricular systolic dysfunction in an urban population. *Lancet*, **350**, 829–833.

10. Morgan, S., Smith, H., Simpson, I. *et al.* (1999) Prevalence and clinical characteristics of left ventricular dysfunction among elderly patients in general practice setting: cross-sectional survey. *British Medical Journal*, **318**, 368–372.

11. Ho, S.F., O'Mahony, M.S., Steward, J.A. *et al.* (2004) Left ventricular systolic dysfunction and atrial fibrillation in older people in the community–a need for screening? *Age and Ageing*, **33** (5), 488–492.

12. Mair, F.S., Crowley, T.S. and Bundred, P.E. (1996) Prevalence, aetiology and management of heart failure in general practice. *British Journal of General Practice*, **46**, 77–79.

13. The Quality Management and Analysis System (2008) Available at www.connectingforhealth.nhs.uk/systemsandservices/gpsupport/qmas.

14. Gnani, S., Gray, J., Khunti, K. and Majeed, A. (2004) Managing heart failure in primary care: first steps in implementing the National Service Framework. *Journal of Public Health*, **26** (1), 42–47.

15. Davie, A.P., Love, M.P. and McMurray, J.J. (1996) Value of ECGs in identifying heart failure due to left ventricular systolic dysfunction. *British Medical Journal*, **313**, 300–301.

16. Jeyaseelan, S., Goudie, B.M., Pringle, S.D. *et al.* (2007) A critical re-appraisal of different ways of selecting ambulatory patients with suspected heart failure for echocardiography. *European Journal of Heart Failure*, **9** (1), 55–61.

17. Khunti, K., Squire, I., Abrams, K.R. and Sutton, A.J. (2004) Accuracy of a 12-lead electrocardiogram in screening patients with suspected heart failure for open access echocardiography: a systematic review and meta-analysis. *European Journal of Heart Failure*, **6** (5), 571–576.

18. Fuat, A., Hungin, A.P. and Murphy, J.J. (2003) Barriers to accurate diagnosis and effective management of heart failure in primary care: qualitative study. *British Medical Journal*, **326**, 196.

19. Hobbs, F.D., Jones, M.I., Allan, T.F. *et al.* (2000) European survey of primary care physician perceptions on heart failure diagnosis and management (Euro-HF). *European Heart Journal*, **21** (22), 1877–1887.

20. Goudie, B.M., Jarvis, R.I., Donnan, P.T. *et al.* (2007) Screening for left ventricular systolic dysfunction using GP-reported ECGs. *British Journal of General Practice*, **57**, 191–195.

21. Lim, T.K., Collinson, P.O., Celik, E. *et al.* (2007) Value of primary care electrocardiography for the prediction of left ventricular systolic dysfunction in patients with suspected heart failure. *International Journal of Cardiology*, **115** (1), 73–74.

22. Jensen, M.S., Thomsen, J.L., Jensen, S.E. *et al.* (2005) Electrocardiogram interpretation in general practice. *The Journal of Family Practice*, **22** (1), 109–113.

23. Zaphiriou, A., Robb, S., Murray-Thomas, T. *et al.* (2005) The diagnostic accuracy of plasma BNP and NTproBNP in patients referred from primary care with suspected heart failure: results of the UK natriuretic peptide study. *European Journal of Heart Failure*, **7** (4), 537–541.

24. Khunti, K., Hearnshaw, H., Baker, R. and Grimshaw, G. (2002) Heart failure in primary care: qualitative study of current management and perceived obstacles to evidence-based diagnosis and management by general practitioners. *European Journal of Heart Failure*, **4** (6), 771–777.

25. Gillespie, N.D. and Pringle, S. (1998) A pilot study of the role of echocardiography in primary care. *British Journal of General Practice*, **48**, 1182.

26. Khunti, K. (2004) Systematic review of open access echocardiography for primary care. *European Journal of Heart Failure*, **6** (1), 79–83.

27. Francis, C.M., Caruana, L., Kearney, P. *et al.* (1995) Open access echocardiography in management of heart failure in the community. *British Medical Journal*, **310**, 634–636.

28. Swedberg, K., Cleland, J., Dargie, H. *et al.* (2005) Guidelines for the diagnosis and treatment of chronic heart failure: full text (update 2005). The Task Force for the diagnosis and treatment of CHF of the European Society of Cardiology. *European Heart Journal*, **26**, 1115–1140.

29. American College of Cardiology/American Heart Association (2005) Guideline update for the diagnosis and management of chronic heart failure in the adult. *Circulation*, **112**, 154–235.

30. McAlister, F.A., Lawson, F.M., Teo, K.K. and Armstrong, P.W. (2001) Randomised trials of secondary prevention programmes in coronary heart disease: systematic review. *British Medical Journal*, **323**, 957–962.

31. Taylor, S., Bestall, J., Cotter, S. *et al.* (2005) Clinical service organisation for heart failure. *Cochrane Database of Systematic Reviews*, (2), CD002752.

32. Khunti, K., Stone, M., Paul, S. *et al.* (2007) Disease management programme for secondary prevention of coronary heart disease and heart failure in primary care: a cluster randomised controlled trial. *Heart*, **93** (11), 1398–1405.

33. Kenchaiah, S., Evans, J.C., Levy, D. *et al.* (2002) Obesity and the risk of heart failure. *The New England Journal of Medicine*, **347** (5), 305–313.

34. Mohler, E.R. 3rd (2004) Mechanisms of aortic valve calcification. *American Journal of Cardiology*, **94** (11), 1396–1402.

35. Cowell, S.J., Newby, D.E., Prescott, R.J. *et al.* (2005) Scottish Aortic Stenosis and Lipid Lowering Trial, Impact on Regression (SALTIRE) Investigators. A randomized trial of intensive lipid-lowering therapy in calcific aortic stenosis. *The New England Journal of Medicine*, **352**, 2389–2397.

36. Moura, L.M., Ramos, S.F., Zamorano, J.L. *et al.* (2007) Rosuvastatin affecting aortic valve endothelium to slow the progression of aortic stenosis. *Journal of the American College of Cardiology*, **49** (5), 554–561.

37. Boon, A., Cheriex, E., Lodder, J. and Kessels, F. (1997) Cardiac valve calcification: characteristics of patients with calcification of the mitral annulus or aortic valve. *Heart*, **78** (5), 472–474.

10

The role of the specialist nurse

Sinéad P. McKee

Stirling Royal Infirmary, Livilands Gate, Stirling

Key messages

- Heart failure nurses are specialist practitioners who treat patients holistically, based on national and locally recommended guidelines.

- They are trained to understand and to address the specific needs of older patients.

- Specialist nurses are ideally placed to coordinate primary and secondary care services.

10.1   Introduction

The underutilization of evidence-based therapies for the management of heart failure has been well documented during recent years [1–5]. Even when therapies are used appropriately, many patients remain symptomatic and at high risk of repeated hospitalization [6]. Deterioration in other conditions such as cardiac ischaemia and renal impairment is a common reason why patients with heart failure are admitted to hospital [7].

The management of heart failure is multifaceted, and requires significant efforts by patients and health care providers alike to manage the condition optimally. In order to facilitate this, the number of specialist nurses involved in the management of heart failure has increased dramatically during the past decade. A specially trained heart

---

A Practical Guide to Heart Failure in Older People, Edited by C Ward and M D Witham
© 2009 John Wiley & Sons, Ltd

failure nurse is an important health care professional, fundamental to the success of any heart failure management programme [8]. These nurses work in primary and secondary care, and their role varies depending on locally agreed policies. They make a significant impact on the management of patients with heart failure.

The availability of heart failure services varies widely throughout Europe and North America. Advanced practice nurses with specialist qualifications and experience manage dedicated heart failure clinics in the USA [9]. The number of such specialist clinics has rapidly increased during the past decade [10]. Of the 673 hospitals in 43 countries who responded to a questionnaire survey, 426 (63%) had a heart failure management programme, half of which ($n = 205$) were located in an outpatient clinic. In the UK, a combination of hospital- and home-based programmes was common (75%). The majority of programmes included physical examination, diagnostic tests, drug titration, patient education and telephone consultation. The health professionals involved varied between countries, but most programmes (89%) involved nurses and physicians. Multidisciplinary teams were active in 56% of all programmes.

Managing older patients with heart failure presents more specific challenges. Many have comorbidity which complicates their management and negatively affects their outcome. Cognitive impairment – even if only mild – can result in poor adherence with medication and self-management strategies and a subsequent deterioration in symptoms. Social isolation and low mood – factors which are common in older patients – can also exacerbate nonadherence with recommended treatment.

In this chapter we will outline the evidence to support the role of specialist nurses in heart failure management and multidisciplinary liaison. Difficulties with adherence and cognitive impairment will also be discussed. Finally, lifestyle issues and self-care strategies will be considered.

10.2   The role of the specialist nurse

Qualified specialist nurses need to not only have a comprehensive understanding of the mechanism of heart failure and its management, but also a diverse mix of skills including advanced clinical assessment and excellent communication, with an ability to work as an autonomous practitioner in challenging settings [8]. An experienced nurse qualified to degree level with experience in cardiology/coronary care nursing and further specialist training is ideally placed to develop this role. Opportunities for their continuing education is essential for them to continue to deliver evidence-based care, and this is increasingly available, certainly in the UK. Experts have suggested that a formal university-based education programme should be completed by all specialist nurses who manage patients with heart failure [9] in order to prepare them for this role. To maintain knowledge and skills, clinical supervision should be provided on a regular basis; this will ensure that specialist nurses remain confident and competent in their role. Lack of updates of clinical competence or staff burnout may jeopardise quality and ultimately have a negative impact on patients.

In most health boards, specialist nurses adhere to protocols for altering medication regimes as clinically indicated [9]. This is an important part of heart failure management, and increases the nurses' scope of practice. It is essential however, that strategies are in place to regularly review the protocols to take into consideration emerging changes in practice, and in so doing continue to deliver evidence-based care. It is equally important that regular service evaluation is carried out and changes implemented as required to maintain high standards of care.

A recent study of predominantly older patients with many comorbidities, suggested that patients and carers anticipated a holistic approach to care with service providers considering not only medication but also psychosocial, spiritual and family needs [11]. Whilst medication is imperative for symptom control and prevention of disease progression, the other factors are equally important. The specialist nurse is in a position to refer to a more appropriate professional to address these issues as required.

Drug titration

The use of drugs in the management of heart failure is discussed in Chapter 6. The underutilization of many of these drugs has been well documented. Traditionally, patients discharged from hospital with a diagnosis of heart failure remained on the same doses of medication with little or no change until follow-up in the outpatient clinic, or until they re-presented to hospital with further decompensation. In recent years, as part of their developing role, heart failure nurses have been integrally involved in the initiation and titration of many of these drugs using locally agreed protocols.

Regular review can be provided by the specialist nurse to ensure that regular blood chemistry monitoring is carried out and further medication adjustments can be made as required. Drug side effects can also be detected and appropriate changes made. Although the therapeutic approach to heart failure in older people is similar to that in younger patients, treatment should be applied cautiously. Reduced doses may be necessary in some patients due to the effects of age on the pharmacokinetic and pharmacodynamic properties of cardiovascular drugs, and also because of renal dysfunction [12]. Furthermore, introducing a complex and changing medication regime can be difficult for older patients to adhere to.

To facilitate drug titration in the UK, a system of supplementary prescribing has evolved (Health and Social Care Act 2001; www.opsi.gov.uk/acts/acts 2001). This government directive has extended prescribing responsibilities to professionals other than doctors, including specialist nurses. It is intended to improve care by providing patients with a more efficient access to medicines. Supplementary prescribing allows specialist heart failure nurses to initiate medical therapy as well as to adjust and optimise therapies. Similar changes have been implemented worldwide. For example, in Sweden, prescribing by nurses was introduced in 1994, while in Canada and some parts of Australia support for nurses to develop a prescribing role exists in rural areas and areas where there is a shortage of doctors [13]. In the United States, advanced practice nurses who carry out heart failure clinics are also able to prescribe. As with supplementary prescribing in the UK, the overall aim is to improve access to treatments for all patients.

The benefits of specialist nurses' involvement in heart failure management

Prior to specialist nurses' involvement, the care of patients with heart failure was often fragmented and the follow-up inconsistent. In one qualitative study, patients and carers described their care as 'professionally led' and not a partnership approach [11]. This study also highlighted continuity of care as an important factor for patients: seeing a different doctor at each appointment resulted in discontent. This is an issue which can be addressed if the same health care professional – for example, the specialist nurse – sees the patient at each visit.

A number of randomized controlled trials have been reported in recent years supporting the role of specialist nurses to facilitate the care of patients with heart failure. A landmark US study [14] demonstrated that they had a positive impact on rates of hospital readmission, cost of care and quality of life within 90 days of hospital discharge in a group of high-risk (age ≥ 70 years) patients with chronic heart failure. Using a nurse-led multidisciplinary intervention, patients and their families were educated with regards to the management of heart failure, the medications were optimized, a specific diet was recommended (including salt and fluid restriction), and social needs were assessed as part of the discharge plan. The patients were followed-up with a combination of clinic visits, home visits by the nurse specialist and telephone follow-up. The control group received routine follow-up.

Although a 90-day follow-up for patients with heart failure is a rather short time frame, the study did have some important findings. Survival without readmission was achieved in 91 of the 142 patients in the intervention group, compared to 75 of 140 in the control group (64% versus 54%, $p = 0.09$). There were 94 readmissions in the control group compared to 53 in the treatment group (risk ratio 0.56; $p = 0.02$). The number of readmissions due to decompensated heart failure was significantly reduced by 56.2% in the treatment group (54 versus 24; $p = 0.04$). The reduction in hospital admissions directly resulted in a reduced total cost of care per patient in the treatment group, while contributing to an improved quality of life.

Benefits were also demonstrated for a combination of education about self-management plus a nurse-led heart failure clinic when compared to usual care [15]. Although no difference in mortality was detected at one year, the mean time to readmission was longer in the intervention group than in the control group (141 days versus 106 days; $p < 0.05$) and the number of days in hospital was fewer (4.2 versus 8.2; $p = 0.07$). The follow-up was patient-initiated, and so depended on patients having a good knowledge of their condition, of self-care strategies, and of what to do if the symptoms increased. Even though they were educated regarding their condition, this may not necessarily translate into action when symptoms deteriorate. Translating this model into practice may therefore be less successful than a service which offers routine follow-up with the option for patients to contact the nurse by telephone between review appointments if required.

A multidisciplinary home-based intervention including routine visiting and telephone follow-up by a cardiac specialist nurse was also successful [16]. During a six-month follow-up period, there were more hospital admissions in the control group (129 versus 77, $p = 0.02$), with 50% of readmissions in both groups being due to a deterioration in heart failure symptoms. More of the intervention group remained event-free (38 versus 51, $p = 0.04$), there were fewer unscheduled read-missions in the treatment group (68 versus 118, $p = 0.03$), and for those who were readmitted fewer days were spent in hospital (460 versus 1173, $p = 0.02$), resulting in a reduction in hospital costs. Early clinical deterioration was evident in 40% of patients visited at home within two weeks of discharge, despite being clinically stable at discharge. On questioning and following tablet counts, 22% of the intervention group were not complying with their medication regime. Furthermore, 90% of the patients were unaware of the importance of fluid and salt restriction. Intervention by the nurse specialist to encourage patients to comply with treatment and develop strategies to monitor symptoms and titrate medication was applied and had a direct effect on the primary endpoint.

- Early post-discharge home visits by specialist nurses result in fewer hospital readmissions.

- All-cause readmissions, including those for decompensated heart failure, are reduced when specialist nurses are involved in patient care.

- Patients who have been under the care of a specialist nurse, but have nevertheless been hospitalized, spend fewer days in hospital than those who have not.

The inclusion criteria for this study stipulated that all subjects should be managed by a cardiologist, and were therefore more likely to be optimally managed. This is not however representative of the management of older heart failure patients in the UK, as the majority are not looked after by cardiologists [2]. The timing of the home visit remains debatable as half of the intervention group had died, were readmitted or had symptoms of clinical deterioration when visited within two weeks, despite being stable at discharge. This, along with the fact that half of the study population was admitted for non-heart failure causes, highlights the complexity of heart failure and underlines the difficulties faced by health care staff.

The first UK study involving nurse specialists in the management of heart failure was carried out in Glasgow [17]. A total of 165 patients (mean age 75 years; range 51–93 years) admitted with heart failure were randomly assigned to the control group with follow-up in accordance with clinical routine at that time ($n = 81$) or to specialist nurse intervention ($n = 84$). The intervention consisted of a review prior to hospital discharge, home visits after two days, three further visits during the first six weeks, and four further visits during the 12-month follow-up period, with intervening telephone calls. Additional follow-up was arranged if required, and patients and their family were encouraged to use the telephone helpline if necessary. Medications were adjusted and titrated according to agreed protocols, blood biochemistry was monitored, and patient education with regard to treatment, non-pharmacological issues and self-care strategies was ongoing throughout the study.

At hospital discharge, more patients in the intervention group were started on ACE inhibitors (65 versus 53%). Mortality in the two groups was similar (30%, $n = 50$). By the primary endpoint, fewer patients in the intervention group had an event (31 versus 43, hazard ratio (HR) = 0.61, CI 0.38–0.96). Death or readmissions for all causes was reduced by 28% (HR = 0.72, CI 0.49–1.04) in the intervention group compared to the controls. The risk of hospital admission with decompensated heart failure was significantly reduced by 62% (HR = 0.38, CI 0.19–0.76) in the intervention group. For patients who were readmitted with deteriorating heart failure, those in the intervention group spent fewer days in hospital (mean 3.43 versus 7.46 days, $p = 0.005$) compared to the control group.

The results of this study showed that intervention by specialist nurses resulted in a considerable reduction in the risk of hospital admission with decompensated heart failure. It was however, a labour-intensive study, and although not discussed it is likely that a reduction in hospital admissions would recoup some of the costs of delivering the service. Indeed, when Stewart *et al.* [18] explored the economic consequence of delivering a nurse-led service for managing heart failure post discharge, they showed that such a service, as well as reducing hospital admissions and improving quality of life, simultaneously decreased overall costs and contributed to a more efficient health care system.

10.3 Clinic-based versus home-based service

There is evidence to support specialist nurses based both in primary care, carrying out home visits, and in a secondary care setting holding clinics. Patients are seen by a specialist nurse during their admission, patient education is commenced, and follow-up arranged depending on what is available locally. The titration of medications and ongoing education is provided as part of the follow-up, regardless of where the patients are seen.

Many clinics are nurse-led, with patients seeing the same specialist nurse at each visit, and such continuity of care is favoured by many patients [11]. Other clinics operate with medical staff and a specialist nurse reviewing the patient, carrying out investigations as required and a management plan devised in a 'one-stop' clinic. This type of clinic is beneficial to patients who may have difficulty attending several different appointments, or if transport is a problem. It may, however, be arduous for older frail patients, especially if it requires attendance at hospital for a prolonged period of time.

A clinic-based service has many advantages. For example, if investigations are required, such as chest X-ray or echocardiography, they can be organized to coincide with the clinic appointments and, if the results are available, the patient can be informed immediately. In theory there should be easier access to cardiologists and other physicians, thereby providing rapid access for advanced treatment such as intravenous diuretics without admission to hospital [19]. Patients' medical records are more easily available for clinic appointments, which is clearly beneficial. From a service provider's perspective, it is more economical to offer a clinic-based service, as a specialist nurse can see more patients in a clinic session without the additional time and cost of travelling. However, for many older patients, or for those with mobility problems, it may not be feasible to attend hospital-based clinics. The timing of clinics can often cause problems for older patients who have carers coming to their home to assist with activities of daily living. If the clinic is early in the morning, the patient's routine is disrupted and they may miss their carer – for many patients this may be the only social contact they have throughout the day. Clinics late in the afternoon may cause the same problems, and additionally patients may be too tired to attend. Many patients fail to attend clinic appointments without giving any notification.

For patients who have advanced heart failure, a hospital-based clinic service is not ideal; it is preferable to review them in their own home, and in some areas health care providers have opted to provide a home-based service. Specialist nurses can be involved in the care of a range of patients, including those on a palliative trajectory and patients who are frail and/or older, many of whom find attending clinics very arduous. Many patients simply do not like attending hospital and may benefit from home visits. In a cohort of patients with heart failure, those from socially deprived areas in Scotland had less ongoing contact with their general practitioners compared to those from affluent areas [20]. Rather, they preferred to attend Accident and Emergency departments with acute episodes of heart failure symptoms. It may be reasonable to suggest that this cohort of patients would be less likely to attend hospital clinics and may therefore benefit from domiciliary visits in order to optimise their management.

Specialist nurses can, within reason, make home visits at a time that is convenient for the patient. There is an option to coordinate visits with family or carers who wish to be involved, or with the multidisciplinary team. Care in the patient's own home is delivered in a more comfortable, non-intimidating environment [12] than that provided at a clinic. In addition, the specialist nurse is able to make a more realistic assessment of the social circumstances and possible problems with noncompliance, and address these accordingly.

Unfortunately, home visits are time-consuming and may not be suited to all areas; moreover, there is limited access to support from cardiologists or other physicians. If investigations are required other than blood tests, patients will need to attend the hospital, and so there may be a delay in carrying out investigations and obtaining results. Furthermore, the specialist nurse will not have access to the patient's medical notes in the community.

In recent years, home telemonitoring has been considered as an adjunct to heart failure management strategies. There is some evidence to support this method of monitoring patients [21], but it is complex and involves the use of technology which may further complicate management for patients. Its transferability into practice, particularly for older patients, remains unclear.

In many cases the geographical layout of the area will dictate what service is more economical for the health care provider. While a home-based service is suited to an urban area, it may not be cost-effective in rural areas where the nurse would spend lengthy periods driving between visits. Hence, a clinic-based service may be better suited to such an area. A combination of clinic and home-based service may be available in some areas, depending on the needs of the patient. This model would service the needs of patients at different stages of the disease trajectory. Patients could be offered an appointment at the clinic to be reviewed by the specialist nurse. If they were unable to attend clinics, then a home visit could be offered. If the infrastructure is correct, care can be delivered effectively through hospital-based clinics, in the patients' own homes, or by using a combination of approaches.

Whichever model is used, a discharge strategy must be incorporated. When patients are on optimum tolerated doses of evidence-based medications, are clinically stable and have a good understanding of their condition, they can be discharged back to the care of their GP. Both, the patient and the GP should be given the option to contact the specialist nurse if symptoms deteriorate, and a review can then be arranged. By discharging stable patients, resources can be directed to other patients whose care is not yet optimized.

10.4   Multidisciplinary team liaison

Specialized heart failure nurses play a pivotal role in coordinating programmes of care to ensure optimal discharge and ongoing management of patients with heart failure. Multidisciplinary collaboration should be encouraged to provide a wide range of services and expertise to these patients. Clear referral pathways ensure optimal use of the different health care professionals.

The role of the pharmacist in patient education is important. In some localities, where a gap in service provision for patients with heart failure exists, pharmacists are involved in the titration of drugs and patient education in the same way as specialist nurses. However, the success of this strategy is unclear. One study assessed the impact of drug review, symptom management and lifestyle advice by community pharmacists to patients discharged from hospital following an admission with heart failure [22]. Patients in the intervention group were reviewed and educated by community pharmacists on two occasions following discharge, but the pharmacist did not titrate the drug doses. There was a trend towards an increase in emergency readmissions in the intervention group compared to the control group (134 versus 112, $p = 0.28$). Furthermore, there was no increase in medication compliance in the intervention group, as might have been expected. However, it was acknowledged by the study investigators that the pharmacists involved in the study were not specialists in heart failure management. Although the results clearly do not support community pharmacists in a role similar to that of the specialist nurse, their input in conjunction with specialist nurses and other health care professionals is essential to improve the patients' knowledge of medication and adherence. It is important that the content of information given to patients and their carers is consistent, especially when different health professionals are involved in its delivery.

Good communication and relations between primary and secondary care staff is essential. Locally agreed management guidelines, including referral pathways developed by primary and secondary care staff, will be beneficial for all practitioners involved in the management of heart failure. Unambiguous prompt correspondence following clinic consultations and discharge is necessary. In one area, hospital-based pharmacists indicated on immediate discharge letters the reason for starting or discontinuing drugs, and this information was found to be very useful for GPs [23].

Specialist nurses have an important role to play in bridging the gap between primary and secondary care. An established network provides support for practitioners while facilitating optimum care for patients. For specialist nurses based in the community, this important link allows continuing clinical assessment, appropriate titration of drugs and patient education with the benefit of support from secondary care colleagues as required.

Primary care staff have a greater awareness of the patient's social and domestic situations [24], and are clearly pivotal to their management. However, it is likely that the specialist nurse, in conjunction with the GP and their staff, will facilitate the patient's care and see them on a regularly basis with involvement of the multidisciplinary team as required. As the heart failure trajectory progresses towards a palliative stage, input from the primary care multidisciplinary team will enhance the patient's journey.

10.5   Specific issues affecting older patients

Cognitive impairment

Impaired cognition is a robust indicator of disease progression and/or concurrent cerebrovascular disease, both of which result in premature mortality [25]. Impaired cognition is common in patients with chronic heart failure, and independently predicts a poor outcome; even mild cognitive impairment can have a negative impact on patient outcome. This presents a challenge to specialist nurses, as well as to other health care professionals involved with these patients, as they are less likely to understand or adhere to the self-care strategies aimed at improving their symptoms.

When patients are admitted to hospital with acute heart failure, the priority is to treat their clinical symptoms. A detailed psychological assessment is generally not carried out and, as a result, mild or even moderate cognitive impairment may be missed. A routine screening for cognitive impairment of patients with chronic heart failure has been studied [25], and this is something that specialist nurses could introduce in conjunction with physicians. Undetected cognitive impairment can result in a deterioration of symptoms as well as causing patients to become withdrawn, resulting in increased levels of depression and anxiety [26].

Social isolation is an important factor in the management of older patients with heart failure, and has been reported as a problem that intensifies stress levels after discharge from hospital [19]. Every effort should be made to address this problem by involving the multidisciplinary team to maximise social service input and ameliorate these feelings for patients. Meeting the patient prior to discharge, as well as an early clinic- or home-based follow-up, is also likely to go some way to ameliorating these concerns.

Compliance and adherence to management advice

Adherence to all aspects of heart failure management will improve symptoms and quality of life, as well as reducing hospital admissions. The precipitating factor for admission to hospital with acute heart failure in 22.2% ($n = 795$) of all patients admitted was nonadherence to prescribed treatment [27], with men more often being nonadherent to medication than women. There was no reference in this study to adherence to non-pharmacological management issues, which are equally important. It may be reasonable to suggest that if patients were not adherent to medication regimes, they may not have adhered to self-care management strategies either.

Complex medication regimes are the cornerstone of heart failure management, but are likely to contribute to the problem of nonadherence. Adherence to medication can be measured by carrying out tablet counts or monitoring blood samples (e.g. serum digoxin or serum ACE activity [28]), but this is neither practical nor economically viable as a routine strategy. Cline *et al.* [29] demonstrated the difficulties with adherence in a small study of older patients (mean age 79) with heart failure. Nonadherence with prescribed medication was common, with only one in four patients being adherent one month after receiving detailed education. The authors believed polypharmacy to be an important contributory factor to non-adherence rather than patient age. A significant number of patients also continued to take medication which had been discontinued during their hospital stay. This may be the result of 'repeat prescription practice' and poor communication between secondary and primary care staff on discharge, and highlights an area where the involvement of specialist nurses could pre-empt such occurrences.

The authors concluded this study by suggesting one strategy to improve adherence, namely the use of simplified medication regimes aimed at reducing polypharmacy. Yet, specialist nurses work in an era where optimising medication in accordance with guidelines is practised, and which is the basis of service evaluation. It is therefore important to assess each individual patient and their circumstances, and tailor care to their needs.

Patients often have a limited understanding of their medications. For example, many patients know the names of their tablets but do not know what they are for [30, 31]. More alarming is the fact that many patients were unable to identify the difference between drug side effects and symptoms of heart failure decompensation [30]. In clinical practice, this is concerning as patients may not know when to seek help. The specialist nurses – and also the pharmacist – can and do advise patients about the actions and side effects of their medications and the appropriate action to take if any adverse effects occur.

The patient's partner or main carers have been shown to have an important role in helping them adhere to their treatment [31]. In this study, one-third of patients managed their medication independently, one-third received reminders from their carer, and one-third relied totally on their carer. In order to adhere to medications, patients identified two main strategies: (i) a routine for taking medication; and (ii) a back-up or some type of aide memoire, for example a visual cue. The authors identified the development of management strategies as a fundamental part of living with chronic disease. Patients in this study identified taking medication as something that they had to learn. Some patients reported what the authors referred to as 'low concordance': deliberately not taking diuretics when going to a social event where they were unsure of the location of toilets. Medication such as diuretics can have a negative impact on the quality of life, and it is therefore important that patients are advised on how to take these drugs in a manner that is compatible with their daily routine. A further example of 'low concordance' was highlighted: if patients were disrupted from their normal routine, they were more likely to unintentionally omit their tablets [31]. This emphasises the importance of having a routine as a strategy for taking medication, and should be highlighted to patients and their carers. These strategies can also be used by patients to facilitate the ordering of prescriptions. If patients are taking numerous medications, they will need to order prescriptions regularly to maintain an adequate supply. Medication supplies running out at different times can be avoided by the coordinated efforts of patients, GPs and their receptionists, specialist nurses and pharmacists.

It is difficult to measure adherence with all aspects of heart failure management. Many patients may give what they think is the appropriate answer when questioned, for example regarding fluid intake. Providing patients with education and advice does not necessarily improve adherence, but it will help if patients have a better understanding of their condition and treatment. The specialist nurse can reinforce information at each visit in order to improve compliance. Particular emphasis should be placed on patients who are socially isolated [28], on older patients, and on those who are well known not to adhere to therapy. There is, however, conflicting information in the literature regarding adherence by those who are older. Some studies report older patients as being more adherent to medication [32, 33], perhaps because they are more likely to be provided with medication aides, whereas another study reported them as being less compliant than their younger counterparts [29]. It is difficult to know how accurately research studies reflect heart failure management, as older patients and/or patients with dementia are often excluded from heart failure studies [34]. Furthermore, patients who participate in research studies are more likely to be motivated to manage their condition and may comply with management simply because they are participating in such a study.

Family and carer support

Providing support for family and carers is an important role for the specialist nurse. If a helpline facility is available, the family or carers should be encouraged to use it to seek general information, advice and support. Social services can also be involved in providing support, both practical and financial. There are many cardiac support groups throughout the country that provide various methods of support, including emotional and social support, information and education [3–5]. Specialist nurses are encouraged to be aware of what is available and to disseminate this information to families and carers.

Specialist nurses play an important part in providing support for patients and their families [35]. In many cases, the presence of the specialist nurse gives reassurance and security to patients. In this study there was also evidence of the patients and families having an emotional dependence on the specialist nurse. While this is clearly beneficial, and highlights the importance of the nurse specialist to the patients and families, it also emphasises the importance of the nurse establishing boundaries and of providing debriefing support.

10.6 End of life care

Heart failure is a chronic condition with a varying disease trajectory. However, the challenge for specialist nurses is to provide care with hope and optimism while maintaining a sense of realism [35]. They can exercise their role in improved symptom control, communication and supporting patients and their families when dealing with end of life issues. In one study, the authors noted that nurse specialists were sought out by patients and their families to interpret information and assist in decision making, especially with regards to resuscitation [35]. Preferred place of care should be discussed with the patient and family. Continuity of care throughout the illness will improve the rapport between the patient and specialist nurse, and should make such topics less challenging to approach. Extrapolating general palliative care to the needs of patients with heart failure using a multidisciplinary approach is recommended [3–5]. These issues are discussed further in Chapter 14.

10.7 Specialist nurses and education

Patient education

Many patients think heart failure means 'heart attack' or 'cardiac arrest' [36]. So, it is important to explain to the patient and their carer what heart failure is and what it is not, as well as to outline the cause of the heart failure and the treatment options and prognosis. It is important to be honest and to avoid giving false hope. As there is no cure for heart failure in most cases, optimum symptom control and prevention of disease progression is the objective of management. This should be made clear to the patient and their carers. At the outset, it is essential to help patients understand that they have a key role to play in the management of their condition – it is not just about taking the tablets! There are many areas of their management in which they can be involved (see Chapter 13).

Good communication between the specialist nurse and the patient are essential to empower the latter to be involved in their own management [36]. However, this can be difficult due to a variety of barriers, especially in those who are older. Barriers to open communication may include functional limitations (visual and hearing loss [37]), cognitive impairment [11, 37] or the adoption of denial as a coping strategy [11]. It is important to differentiate between these so that patients can be provided with information according to their needs. In older patients, it may be necessary to reiterate information due to both cognitive impairment and functional limitations.

Barriers to learning have also been identified in the literature. These include comorbidity (especially in older patients), misconceptions, a high prevalence of anxiety and depression, and social isolation – particularly in those who do not have a partner or carer [37]. Overcoming these barriers is extremely challenging for all members of the primary care team, including the specialist nurse. In order to effectively educate patients, strategies to deal with these issues are required, and this includes assessing each patient individually, providing tailored education and establishing a partnership approach with patients.

The timing of education for patients and carers is important, as too much information given at the wrong time may be detrimental. In one UK-based qualitative study [30], some patients felt that information was given to them at an inappropriate time, for example when they had just been told of their diagnosis and they were too shocked to absorb anything further. Planned education in a staged approach, sensitive to the patients' needs and stage of acceptance, will be advantageous.

Verbal information regarding heart failure and its management should be supplemented with written information for the patients and their carers to read, and should be provided in an easily understood format. The British Heart Foundation [38], the Scottish Intercollegiate Guidelines Network [39] and other organizations have each published various booklets providing basic information for patients. However, a more comprehensive and widely available book by Cowie [40] relates the information in an easily understood manner, provides unambiguous explanations of normal heart function, what heart failure is, and its causes, diagnosis and treatment. The book also provides a list of useful contacts for further information. Based on the present author's experience, both carers and patients with heart failure alike have viewed this book very positively.

Education for the multidisciplinary team

As an expert practitioner in the management of heart failure, the specialist nurse is suitably placed to improve the knowledge and skills of other members of the team, and should be used as a resource for the other professionals. A rolling education programme covering all areas of heart failure management should be offered for primary and secondary care staff. The specialist nurse can be influential in coordinating this, in conjunction with other experts.

References

1. Blue, L., Lang, E., McMurray, J.J.V. *et al.* (2001) Randomised controlled trial of specialist nurse intervention in heart failure. *British Medical Journal*, **323**, 715–718.
2. McKee, S.P., Leslie, S.J., LeMaitre, J.P. *et al.* (2003) Management of chronic heart failure due to systolic left ventricular dysfunction by cardiologist and non-cardiologist physicians. *The European Journal of Heart Failure*, **5**, 549–555.
3. American College of Cardiology/American Heart Association (2005) Guideline update for the diagnosis and management of chronic heart failure in the adult. *Circulation*, **112**, 154–235.
4. Swedberg, K., Cleland, J., Dargie, H. *et al.* (2005) Guidelines for the diagnosis and treatment of chronic heart failure. The Task Force for the diagnosis and treatment of CHF of the European Society of Cardiology. *European Heart Journal*, **26**, 1115–1140.
5. Scottish Intercollegiate Guidelines Network (SIGN) (2007) *Management of Chronic Heart Failure. A National Clinical Guideline 95.* Royal College of Physicians, Edinburgh. Available at www.sign.ac.uk.
6. Leslie, S.J. and Imray, E.A. (2005) Chronic heart failure: a review. *The Practitioner*, **249**, 262–275.
7. Berry, C., Murdoch, D.R. and McMurray, J.J.V. (2001) Economics of chronic heart failure. *The European Journal of Heart Failure*, **3**, 283–291.
8. McAlister, F.A., Stewart, S., Ferrua, S. and McMurray, J.J. (2004) Multidisciplinary strategies for the management of heart failure patients at high risk for admission: a systematic review of randomised trials. *Journal of the American College of Cardiology*, **44**, 810–819.
9. Blue, L. and McMurray, J. (2005) How much responsibility should heart failure nurses take? *The European Journal of Heart Failure*, **7**, 351–361.
10. Jaarsma, T., Strömberg, A., De Geest, S. *et al.* (2006) Heart failure management programmes in Europe. *European Journal of Cardiovascular Nursing*, **5**, 197–205.
11. Boyd, K.J., Murray, S.A., Kendall, M. *et al.* (2004) Living with advanced heart failure: a prospective, community based study of patients and their carers. *The European Journal of Heart Failure*, **6**, 585–591.
12. Jaarsma, T. (2005) Inter-professional team approach to patients with heart failure. *Heart*, **91**, 832–838.
13. Courtenay, M., Carey, N. and Burke, J. (2007) Independent extended supplementary nurse prescribers, their prescribing practice and confidence to educate and assess prescribing students. *Education Today*, **27**, 739–747.

14. Rich, M.W., Beckham, V., Wittenberg, C. *et al.* (1995) A multidisciplinary intervention to prevent the readmission of elderly patients with congestive heart failure. *New England Journal of Medicine*, **333**, 1190–1195.

15. Cline, C., Israelsson, B., Willenheimer, R. *et al.* (1998) A cost effective management programme for heart failure reduces hospitalisation. *Heart*, **80**, 442–446.

16. Stewart, S., Marley, J.E. and Horowitz, J.D. (1999) Effects of a multidisciplinary, home-based intervention on readmissions and survival among patients with chronic congestive heart failure: a randomised controlled study. *The Lancet*, **354**, 1077–1083.

17. Blue, L. and McMurray, J.J.V. (2001) A specialist nurse-led, home based intervention in Scotland, in *Improving Outcomes in Chronic Heart Failure. A Practical Guide to Specialist Nurse Intervention* (eds S. Stewart and L. Blue), British Medical Journal, London. pp. 79–93.

18. Stewart, S., Blue, L., Walker, A. *et al.* (2002) An economic analysis of specialist heart failure nurses management in the U.K. *European Heart Journal*, **23**, 1369–1378.

19. Yu, D.S.F., Thompson, D.R. and Lee, D.T.F. (2006) Disease management programmes for older people with heart failure: crucial characteristics which improve post discharge outcomes. *European Heart Journal*, **27**, 596–612.

20. McAlister, F.A., Murphy, N.F., Simpson, C.R. *et al.* (2004) Influence of socio-economic deprivation on the primary care burden and treatment of patients with a diagnosis of heart failure in general practice in Scotland: population based study. *British Medical Journal*, **328**, 1110–1113.

21. Cleland, J.G.F., Louis, A.A., Rigby, A.S. *et al.* (2005) Non-invasive home telemonitoring for patients with heart failure at high risk of recurrent admission and death. *Journal of the American College of Cardiology*, **45**, 1654–1664.

22. Holland, R., Brooksby, I., Lenaghan, E. *et al.* (2007) Effectiveness of visits from community pharmacists for patients with heart failure: HeartMed randomised controlled trial. *British Medical Journal*, **334**, 1098–1104.

23. Fuat, A. (2005) Bridging the treatment gap: the primary care perspective. *Heart*, **91**, 35–38.

24. Ward, C. (2004) The quality of life in heart failure. Just talking about it will not make it better. *The European Journal of Heart Failure*, **6**, 535–537.

25. McLennan, S.N., Pearson, S.A., Cameron, J. and Stewart, S. (2006) Prognostic importance of cognitive impairment in chronic heart failure patients: does specialist management make a difference? *The European Journal of Heart Failure*, **8**, 494–501.

26. Lackey, J. (2006) Congestive heart failure and cognitive dysfunction, in *Issues in Heart Failure Nursing* (eds C. Jones and M. Cowie), M&K Publishing, Cumbria, pp. 63–71.

27. Nieminen, M.S., Harjola, V., Hochadel, M. *et al.* (2008) Gender related differences in patients presenting with acute heart failure. Results from EuroHeart Failure Survey II. *The European Journal of Heart Failure*, **10**, 140–148.

28. van der Wal, M.H.L., Jaarsma, T. and van Veldhuisen, D.J. (2005) Non-compliance in patients with heart failure: how can we manage it? *The European Journal of Heart Failure*, **7**, 5–17.

29. Cline, C.M.J., Björck-Linné, A.K., Israelsson, B.Y.A. *et al.* (1999) Non-compliance and knowledge of prescribed medication in elderly patients with heart failure. *The European Journal of Heart Failure*, **1**, 145–149.

30. Field, K., Ziebland, S., McPherson, A. and Lehman, R. (2006) 'Can I come off the tablets now?' A qualitative analysis of heart failure patients' understanding of their medication. *Family Practice*, **23**, 624–630.

31. Reid, M., Clark, A., Murdoch, D.L. *et al.* (2006) Patients strategies for managing medication for chronic heart failure. *International Journal of Cardiology*, **109**, 66–73.

32. Monane, M., Bohn, R.L., Gurwitz, J.H. *et al.* (1994) Non-compliance with congestive heart failure therapy in the elderly. *Archives of Internal Medicine*, **154**, 433–437.

33. Michalsen, A., König, G. and Thimme, W. (1998) Preventable causative factors leading to hospital admission with decompensated heart failure. *Heart*, **80**, 437–441.

34. McMurray, J.J.V. and Stewart, S. (2002) The burden of heart failure. *European Heart Journal Supplements*, **4**, D50–D58.

35. Davidson, P., Paull, G., Rees, D. *et al.* (2005) Activities of home-based heart failure nurse specialists: a modified narrative analysis. *American Journal of Critical Care*, **14**, 429–432.

36. Cowie, M.R. and Kirby, M. (2003) *Managing Heart Failure in Primary Care – A Practical Guide*, Bladon, Oxfordshire.

37. Strömberg, A. (2005) The crucial role of patient education in heart failure. *The European Journal of Heart Failure*, **7**, 363–369.

38. British Heart Foundation (2007) *Living with Heart Failure*. British Heart Foundation, London.

39. Scottish Intercollegiate Guidelines Network (SIGN) (2007) *Chronic Heart Failure for Patients*. Royal College of Physicians, Edinburgh.

40. Cowie, M.R. (2003) *Living with Heart Failure – A Guide for Patients*, Bladon, Oxfordshire.

11

The role of the heart failure specialist

Maheshwar Pauriah, Aaron K.F. Wong and Chim C. Lang

University of Dundee, Ninewells Hospital and Medical School, Dundee

---

Key messages

- Heart failure specialists provide an accessible diagnostic and advice service for hospital- and community-based colleagues.

- The specialist, either local or regional, assesses the suitability of patients for surgical and device therapy interventions.

- Specialists provide an oversight of local heart failure nurses and educational support for professional colleagues.

- Specialists are well placed to develop local treatment guidelines and to coordinate management pathways for heart failure care.

11.1 Introduction

Although the majority of patients with congestive heart failure (CHF) are aged over 65 years, information on this section of the CHF population is limited because clinical trials typically enrol younger patients, and the few population-based studies in older patients with CHF lack detail. Older heart failure patients have many complaints and a poor global health status. Their symptoms are of both cardiac and noncardiac origin, because of the high prevalence of multiple comorbidities, the side effects of

---

A Practical Guide to Heart Failure in Older People, Edited by C Ward and M D Witham
© 2009 John Wiley & Sons, Ltd

medication, and the psychosocial consequences of a chronic, progressive illness. Currently, older CHF patients are mostly cared for by general practitioners (GPs) in the community, and by general physicians, geriatricians or cardiologists when they are hospitalized. Recent data have suggested that there are differences in the diagnostic process and therapeutic management, depending on the professional care providers, and that this can affect the clinical outcome depending on the speciality of the physician responsible for their care [1, 2]. Disease-management programmes supported by heart failure specialists have been proposed and tested to improve the quality of CHF care [3]. In this chapter, we will discuss the role of the heart failure specialist in the management of older CHF patients during the in-hospital phase of care, including the optimization of their medical regimen, the management of clinical deterioration and the evaluation of patients for revascularization and device therapy. We will also discuss the wider role of the specialist with respect to the provision of support for hospital colleagues, for the primary care teams, and for specialist nurses.

11.2   The role of the heart failure specialist

There are very few doctors, outside of tertiary referral centres or academic departments, who devote their time exclusively to the management of patients with heart failure. In the UK, most heart failure specialists are cardiologists who have a special interest in this patient group, but spend only some of their time providing a heart failure service. Increasingly, geriatricians are taking on a similar role. In addition, in the larger group practices, a member of the primary care team will concentrate on treating patients with cardiac problems, including heart failure. Local members of these different groups of specialists usually liaise closely in order to share expertise, knowledge and diagnostic facilities.

The clinical service provided by a hospital-based heart failure specialist normally involves a combination of the care of inpatients, a heart failure clinic and providing advice to colleagues caring for patients on other wards or in the community. In broad terms, however, the different groups of doctors specialising in the management of heart failure patients provide some or all of the following services:

- The provision of a diagnostic service.

- The assessment of patients with symptoms of mixed aetiology.

- The management of patients with acute or worsening heart failure symptoms.

- The management of patients with symptoms resistant to routine treatment.

- The assessment and/or treatment of patients for device therapy or surgical intervention.

- Contributing to the local multidisciplinary care programme.

- The maintenance of clear lines of communication between the heart failure service and primary care.

- Involvement in the provision of palliative care support.

- The development and updating of local treatment guidelines.

In practice, relatively few physicians who offer specialist support for heart failure patients are in a position to offer all of these services, mainly because of constraints imposed by time, geography or finance. Nevertheless, there are in the UK, facilities within each NHS region to fulfil all of the roles listed.

11.3 The provision of a diagnostic service and patient assessment

Doctors working in primary care in most parts of the UK now have access to an echocardiography service for patients with suspected heart failure. However, a common complaint from those working in primary care is that they are unable to interpret some echocardiography reports because of the terminology used. Clearly, in addition to containing a statement of the anatomical/pathological findings and a series of measurements, the report should indicate whether:

- In the light of the information provided with the request form, the findings are consistent with heart failure, or not.

- The findings merit specialist evaluation, for example when there is evidence of valvular pathology.

The heart failure specialist is ideally placed to provide this information.

The diagnosis of heart failure is discussed in detail in Chapter 5. The cut-off point – in echocardiographic terms – between a normal and an abnormal left ventricular ejection fraction (LVEF) is usually accepted as 45%. Inevitably, however, there are some patients who do not fit neatly into having heart failure (i.e. LVEF <45%) or having a functionally normal heart. This is particularly the case with many older patients who have left ventricular (LV) hypertrophy and associated diastolic impairment resulting from hypertension, which is normally accompanied by a preserved LV systolic function (see Chapter 2), but who also have a degree of systolic dysfunction because of concomitant coronary artery disease (see Chapter 4). There are also a number of functionally normal subjects with structurally normal hearts in whom the LVEF is between 40 and 50%. In such cases, heart failure specialists will be expected to 'give a ruling', although in practice when there remains any doubt the patient will be kept under observation for a period or offered a trial of 'heart failure treatment' and assessed with respect to any symptomatic improvement.

Comorbidities are common in patients with heart failure, especially in those who are older (see Chapter 8). This is a common cause of diagnostic difficulty (see Chapter 5) which applies particularly to patients with chronic obstructive pulmonary disease (COPD), anaemia or impaired renal function, although more often the issue is not one of deciding which of two conditions is exclusively responsible for a patient's symptoms but rather to what extent each is contributing. In such situations, the heart failure specialist may be able make an assessment based on available investigations; in others cases, colleagues from other specialities will be involved – both for diagnosis and for shared care of the patient.

11.4   Management of patients with acute or worsening heart failure symptoms

Management of acute heart failure

Most episodes of hospitalization due to heart failure are the result of an exacerbation of CHF or to new onset acute heart failure. Although in the UK at present the heart failure specialist is responsible for the care of the acute phase of the hospitalization of some of these patients, most are under the care of other cardiologists and physicians. Some aspects of the in-hospital management of CHF will therefore be detailed in Chapter 12, which is devoted to the subject of hospitalization.

Patients hospitalized because of heart failure will present with increasing symptoms that include various combinations of exertional dyspnoea, orthopnoea, paroxysmal nocturnal dyspnoea, increasing pitting oedema and sometimes with abdominal pain due to liver congestion. Assessment includes a careful history and physical examination. Routine investigations consist of an ECG, chest X-ray and a biochemical screening that includes the measurement of troponin levels because an acute coronary syndrome (ACS), which sometimes is clinically silent, is a common precipitant of hospitalization.

The initial therapy includes:

- High-flow oxygen.

- Opiates, to relieve the sensation of breathlessness and also act as a pulmonary venodilator. Opiates should always be used in conjunction with an anti-emetic. For older patients they should be used cautiously, but can be up-titrated if needed.

- An intravenous diuretic (furosemide) has been used traditionally to decrease afterload and to promote diuresis.

- Intravenous nitrates are also used; these are vasodilators and decrease both preload and afterload; they also reduce the pulmonary capillary wedge pressure, which is an indirect measurement of the pressure in the left atrium.

- Severe pulmonary oedema unresponsive to conventional medical management may require respiratory support; this can be provided by using continuous positive airways pressure (CPAP) or bilevel positive airways pressure (BiPAP).

- Although noninvasive ventilation induces a more rapid improvement in respiratory distress and metabolic disturbance than does standard oxygen therapy, it has no effect on short-term mortality [4].

- Intubation and ventilation is the next option for patients who are severely acidotic. This option should be discussed carefully with the family and the Intensive Care Unit physicians. Age *per se* should not be a factor in deciding whether ICU care should be provided to a patient.

- Inotropic agents should not be used routinely, but only after the cause of hypotension has been determined.

It is important that patients with acute pulmonary oedema are nursed in a critical care area – a Coronary Care Unit or High-Dependency Unit if at all possible. This will allow health care professionals to titrate vasodilators and other drugs with caution. When the patient has been stabilized, which is usually within the first 24 h, they can be weaned off the venodilators. The diuretics can also be changed from intravenous to oral, and other medications such as angiotensin-converting enzyme (ACE) inhibitors and spironolactone started, if not already prescribed. During the hospital stay, all other pharmacological agents should be optimized. There should be a clear discharge plan and an arranged outpatient visit; nurse specialists will ideally be available for advice in the meantime. There is good evidence to suggest that advice provided by nurse specialists reduces further hospitalizations [5, 6].

The heart failure specialist has a key role to play in assisting with treatment decisions regarding respiratory and inotropic support for severely unwell heart failure patients, and in drawing up protocols for the management of acute heart failure.

Treatment-resistant heart failure

Hospital admissions for acute decompensated heart failure have increased during the past few decades, and are expected to continue to increase. Diuretic resistance may be a feature in a significant proportion of older patients who often have accompanying renal dysfunction, and these patients are considered to have the cardiorenal syndrome. Strategies for overcoming resistance to loop diuretics in patients include increasing the dose size of the loop diuretic; continuous intravenous infusion of the diuretic; or concomitant administration of another diuretic such as metolazone or hydrochlorothiazide (see Chapter 12). The combination strategy with thiazide diuretics may result in significant potassium loss, and therefore there is a need for urea and electrolytes monitoring as well as daily checks of body weight. The recommend weight loss is no more than 1 kg per day. For those patients who fail to respond to the above measures, it is important to ensure that there is no mechanical obstruction such as prostatic hypertrophy. Nephrotoxic drugs (e.g. non-steroidal anti-inflammatory drugs; NSAIDS) should be avoided. When the above measures have been introduced, inotropic agents may be considered if the response has been unsatisfactory. Catecholamine- and phosphodiesterase-based inotropic therapies are effective, but the increased risk of arrhythmogenesis and the increased mortality rates seen in clinical trials limit their use. The experimental agent levosimendan is a positive inotropic agent, but does not increase myocyte calcium concentrations, as do catecholamines or phosphodiesterase inhibitors. Although a positive survival benefit for levosimendan versus dobutamine has been reported, the mortality benefit observed in earlier studies has not been confirmed in recent, larger clinical trials [7].

There are some emerging therapies for acute decompensated heart failure. With almost 30% of patients developing diuretic resistance, treatments with diuretics have a limited success. Hence, if all of the above treatments fail, haemofiltration or ultrafiltration can be used. Early ultrafiltration in acute decompensated heart failure patients with diuretic resistance will not only improve rehospitalization rates but also safely and effectively reduce congestion in these patients [8].

Evidence regarding the potential renal-preserving effects of nesiritide is mixed, and further studies on the efficacy and safety of different doses in heart failure therapy are warranted [9]. Newer therapeutic agents, including vasopressin antagonists and adenosine antagonists, hold promise for the future and clinical trials of these agents are presently under way [10–12].

11.5   Optimization of heart failure treatment

Pharmacological therapy

An important role of the heart failure specialist is to guide GPs and physicians towards an optimal oral drug therapy for CHF. The development of local guidelines based on best evidence is one way in which heart failure specialists can influence the pharmacological management of heart failure. Another important role for the heart failure specialist is in managing those patients in whom drug therapy is less straightforward. Examples include:

- Patients with renal impairment: Careful dose titration may be required, with the specialist and heart failure nurse liaising closely to ensure that the tightrope between heart failure decompensation and worsening renal impairment is successfully negotiated. The heart failure specialist is also likely to have easier access to specialist investigation, for example for renal artery stenosis, and is likely to have more experience of less well used therapies, for example nitrates and hydralazine.

- Patients intolerant of multiple heart failure medications: Similarly, careful titration may be required. Ambiguity sometimes exists as to whether symptoms are truly worsened by medications, for example cough with ACE inhibitors, breathlessness with beta-blockers. The heart failure specialist can provide a useful second opinion on such matters to try and ensure high rates of evidence-based drug use.

- Patients with advanced symptoms requiring multiple medications: The occasional patient may require dual blockade with ACE inhibitors and angiotensin-receptor blockers (ARBs). Patients with advanced CHF may also require digoxin or spironolactone. Such combinations have high side effect rates, especially in older people, and cause biochemical derangement (e.g. hyponatraemia, hyperkalaemia) as well as symptom-related problems such as dizziness. At this point the judgement of the heart failure specialist may be useful in deciding how to balance the benefits of such therapies, with their potential side effects.

The heart failure specialist also provides a conduit for access to recently licensed medications or experimental medications as part of clinical trials, with potential consequent benefits to patients.

Device therapy

In recent years, device therapy has revolutionized the treatment of CHF, and heart failure specialists are now increasingly involved in both the selection and implantation of these devices. Implantation is often technically complex, and patient selection frequently requires sophisticated investigation. The heart failure specialist has an important role in patient selection and liaison with other members of the electrophysiology multidisciplinary team. Clinical practice guideline recommendations on device therapy have been driven by clinical trials that have consistently shown improvements in symptoms and in the quality of life, as well as decreased hospitalization and dramatic improvements in survival in selected groups of patients. The various devices that can be implanted are detailed in the following section.

Pacing for bradycardia

The indications for conventional pacemaker therapy in patients with CHF who are unsuitable for cardiac resynchronization therapy (CRT) or for the implantation of an automated cardioverter defibrillator (see below) are the same as for patients with normal LV function. These can be found in the American College of Cardiology/ American Heart Association guidelines for permanent pacemaker (PPM) implantation [13]. The guidelines also suggest that PPM is indicated in ". . .arrhythmias and other medical conditions that require drugs that result in symptomatic bradycardia. (Level of Evidence: C)" [13]. As right ventricular pacing is associated with LV dyssynchrony, there is emerging evidence that in patients with CHF considered for bradycardia pacing, these patients should be offered CRT or biventricular pacing [14].

Automated implantable cardioverter defibrillator (AICD)

Patients with CHF may die suddenly and unpredictably from an arrhythmia, despite the use of proven medical therapies. Medical therapies such as beta-blockers, ACE inhibitors and spironolactone reduce the incidence of sudden cardiac death (as discussed in other chapters). Various trials have examined the value of the AICD in optimally treated patients in ischaemic and nonischaemic cardiomyopathy. An AICD is a special type of device (similar to a pacemaker) which monitors the cardiac rhythm, although if ventricular fibrillation (VF) or ventricular tachycardia (VT) is detected, then a shock is delivered. The detection of VF/VT is based mainly on the heart rate together with an algorithm detection software designed to reduce the risk of inappropriate shocks due to atrial fibrillation, atrial flutter and sinus tachycardia.

The SCD-HeFT trial randomized optimally treated heart failure patients in whom the LVEF was <35% and who were in NYHA functional classes II or III. Amiodarone had no favourable effect on survival, whereas single-lead, shock-only AICD therapy reduced the overall mortality by 23% [15]. Although there was no upper limit for age, the median age was only 60 years and the interquartile range 50–69 years.

Prior to AICD implantation, all patients must provide their well-informed consent, with all risks and benefits having been explained. The placement of an AICD does not alter cardiac contractility, but merely prevents sudden cardiac death. In patients with severe heart disease, AICD implantation may only change the mode of death from sudden cardiac death (SCD) to death from pump failure. In end-stage cardiac failure, the AICD will continue to shock the dying heart and, in the absence of any reversible causes, it may then be appropriate to switch off the AICD. However, this is a very sensitive issue and should only be undertaken after careful discussion with the patient and family. Such an action should also be performed by an appropriately trained health care professional, usually one who is a member of cardiac department team.

Inappropriate shock remains a problem, although the risk is much less with the newer devices and discriminating algorithms. In skilled hands, about 10% of patients with an ICD will have inappropriate shocks.

Cardiac resynchronization therapy (CRT)

This is a relatively novel therapy where, in patients with left bundle branch block, the left ventricle is activated later than the right ventricle and the septum. This leads to ventricular dyssynchrony that leads to a reduced LVEF, worsening symptoms and mitral regurgitation. Biventricular pacing – which involves the simultaneous pacing of the right and left ventricles – improves the ventricular dyssynchrony and leads to an improved exercise capacity, a decrease in NYHA class, decreased hospitalization and an improved survival. The CARE-HF study [16] demonstrated, in a large randomized controlled trial, the efficacy in improving survival in a carefully selected group of patients with the following criteria:

- Age ≥18 years

- NYHA class III or IV

- 'High standard' pharmacological therapy, including ACE inhibitors or ARBs and aldosterone-receptor blockers (for advanced heart failure)

- LVEF ≤35%

- LV end-diastolic dimension (LVEDD ≥30 mm)

- QRS interval ≥120 ms.

The mean patient age in this study was 66/67 years. While no trials have specifically investigated older patients, there is evidence to suggest that CRT also improves surrogate markers in these patients [17].

The combination of CRT with a defibrillator (CRT-D) is increasingly being used, and patients in whom it is intended to implant such devices should provide their full consent. NYHA class IV is commonly considered to be a contraindication to the use of an AICD, although it can be argued that in selected patients CRT would decrease the NYHA class from IV to III, in which case the implantation of a separate defibrillator coil would improve survival. Currently, some physicians elect to place a defibrillator coil in such patients and, if the NYHA class improves, the CRT is upgraded to a CRT-D using a minimally invasive procedure.

11.6   Treatment of reversible causes of heart failure

Revascularization: percutaneous coronary intervention and coronary artery bypass grafting

Despite the increasing number of older patients presenting with an acute coronary syndrome and CHF (see Chapter 12), these patients are often excluded from randomized clinical trials of percutaneous coronary intervention (PCI). Reasons given for this include the severity and complexity of coronary artery lesions in older patients, which often results in them having fewer direct stenting procedures, and in those who do have stenting a longer X-ray exposure and a higher volume of contrast medium use. Furthermore, the increased risk of stroke and high prevalence of comorbidity in these patients (e.g. anaemia and renal failure) makes them the least attractive subset of patients to evaluate in PCI trials.

Although the clinical merit of revascularization in patients with severe systolic heart failure is unclear, there is increasing data which does suggest that in patients with angina *in addition* to having symptoms of CHF, revascularization either in the form of coronary artery bypass grafting (CABG) or PCI may improve the outcome [18]. However, it should be stressed that the management of older patients with CHF without ischaemic symptoms (but with angiographic evidence of coronary artery disease) is less straightforward. Furthermore, because older patients often present with atypical symptoms, clinical evaluation difficult may be difficult. For example, they may complain of breathlessness as an 'angina equivalent' rather than of chest tightness. Despite this, these patients have a similar three-year cardiac mortality when compared to patients who presented with typical symptoms [19]. There is, however, a reluctance to refer older patients at an early stage for PCI, partly for the reasons noted above and partly because of other concerns, including the worry of major adverse cardiac events (MACE) during and after the procedure, and the risk of procedure-related bleeding, notably in those patients with renal dysfunction.

In contrast, Batchelor and colleagues reported that the procedural risk of PCI in older patients is decreasing [20], while Costa and coworkers showed that PCI with drug-eluting stents was associated with a low incidence of MACE and a comparable in-hospital success rate between patients aged less than 70 years and those who were older [21]. Additionally, in a retrospective analysis, Sukiennik and colleagues showed that older patients who underwent PCI had a high procedural success rate [22]. Nevertheless, it was concluded that advanced age remains the most important prognosticator for in-hospital outcome. In another retrospective analysis, Guo and colleagues described treatment with early PCI as being superior to thrombolysis in older patients presenting with acute myocardial infarction (MI) and cardiogenic shock. A Cox regression analysis also showed early PCI to be an independent prognosticator of mid-term survival [23].

There is, therefore, increasing evidence to suggest that PCI in older patients with CHF is not only safe, but can also be beneficial in that it can relieve angina. However, it should be noted that much of this favourable evidence is derived from non-randomized clinical trials. The role of the heart failure specialist in this situation would be to evaluate the risk and benefits of the procedure on an individual patient basis.

Clearly, additional randomized trials are required to clarify the most appropriate treatment (conservative versus interventional) for patients in different age groups.

With regards to CABG, there is mounting evidence suggesting that it improves the clinical outcome and functional state of patients with CHF [24, 25]. The Coronary Artery Surgery Study [26] conducted during the 1980s demonstrated a superiority of surgery over medical management of patients with impaired LV function and coronary artery disease, with five-year survival being significantly better among surgical patients (68%) than in the medical group (54%). The LV function may improve significantly following revascularization, although functional recovery of the hibernating myocardium (i.e. myocardium which, due to chronic ischaemia, is severely but reversibly impaired) may take several months. (The likelihood of this beneficial outcome is routinely assessed before considering CABG in patients with heart failure by myocardial thallium scanning or dobutamine stress echocardiography.) However, the added risk of stroke and/or postoperative complications due to coexisting conditions must also be considered prior to a patient being considered for bypass surgery.

Valvular surgery

The aetiology of CHF is diverse (see Chapter 4), and surgery is dramatically effective in some patients with a reversible cause, specifically in those cases caused by valvular disease. Before surgery is contemplated, however, patients must be fully assessed and the risk/benefit ratio determined by an expert. While it is important not to deny surgery to groups who might benefit, this is not a 'one size fits all' solution.

Aortic stenosis

The prevalence of aortic stenosis (valve area $\leq 1.2 \, \text{cm}^2$) in the general population increases with age, from 2.5% at 75 years to 8.1% at 85 years. However, with an ageing population the incidence and prevalence of severe AS will inevitably increase (see Chapter 4).

The transvalvular aortic valve gradient (a standard means of assessing the severity of aortic stenosis) depends on the LV function. As the left ventricle fails, the transvalvular gradient will decreases, even with severe aortic stenosis, which in turn makes the assessment of severity more difficult. In this situation, dobutamine stress echocardiography can be used to decide who will benefit most from surgery. In the setting of low-gradient aortic stenosis, surgery seems beneficial for most patients with a LV contractile reserve [27] – that is, those in whom the LV function will respond to an infusion of dobutamine.

There are clear clinical guidelines for the treatment of young and middle-aged patients with aortic stenosis. Such guidelines indicate that, in general, patients with symptomatic stenosis – including most of those with evidence of heart failure – should undergo aortic valve replacement (AVR). In older patients, who most likely will have multiple comorbidities, the risk/benefit ratio is less clear. In fact, community-based studies have shown that only a minority of patients with severe aortic stenosis are referred to tertiary centres to be assessed for surgery [25], which is the only definitive treatment. In skilled surgical centres, the mortality from AVR in older patients is less than 10% [26], whereas for those who refuse surgery – or in whom it is contraindicated – the mortality may be 12-fold higher. Patients should, therefore, be aware of these risks and benefits before making a decision. Age *per se* is not an acceptable contraindication to surgery [28]; for example, Professor Richard DeBakey – one of the pioneers of cardiac surgery – underwent surgery for aortic dissection at the age of 97 and made a good recovery!

Today, approximately 200 000 patients undergo valve replacement worldwide each year, although it is estimated that one-third or more [22] of patients with comparably severe disease do not receive surgery, due either to excessive risk factors and comorbidities or to patient refusal for fear of lifestyle changes after major surgery in older patients. It is important to note, however, that these findings were based on all patients who had attended hospital – it did not exclusively survey patients with heart failure. Consequently, the percentage of older patients with heart failure who do not have surgery would be much higher than the figure quoted above.

Moreover, with an ageing population, this number will increase even further. Recently, percutaneous aortic valve replacement has been shown as feasible, and has attracted great interest and enthusiasm among cardiologists. In fact, two multicentre studies have recently started enrolment in Europe (REVIVE trial) and the US (REVIVAL trial), that should help to determine the future of this revolutionary and promising interventional cardiology procedure.

Mitral regurgitation

During the natural history of valvular mitral regurgitation (MR) (see Chapter 4) the left ventricle is initially hyperdynamic; however, as the degree of MR increases, the ventricle dilates in order to maintain the cardiac output. At this stage, because of the haemodynamic characteristics of MR, the normal indicators of impaired LV function (LVEF <45%; see Chapter 5) are misleading. When the LVEF falls below 60% in the presence of severe MR, the prognosis after surgical correction is worsened

[29]. Hence, those patients in whom MR is associated with symptoms of heart failure should be referred promptly for assessment.

Functional MR commonly occurs secondary to myocardial infarction, and is therefore often associated with a low LVEF [30]. Mitral annuloplasty can be beneficial in improving LV function, but the benefit is usually only temporary and it is not clear at present whether CABG with or without mitral valve replacement is better, there having been no randomized controlled trials to determine this point. The prevention of functional MR is clearly better than surgery, and with growing numbers of patients undergoing PCI to treat an ACS, the role for surgery in the treatment of ischaemic functional MR can be expected to diminish.

11.7 Treatment of concomitant diseases (see also Chapter 8)

Comorbidities often seriously impact on the management of patients with heart failure, the most common being anaemia, renal failure and atrial fibrillation [49].

Anaemia

Anaemia is present in a substantial proportion (15–55%) of the CHF population, depending on the definition of anaemia and severity of the heart disease [31]. Anaemia is independently associated with increased morbidity and impaired prognosis [32]; the exact mechanism by which this occurs is as yet undetermined, but a multifactorial aetiology has been proposed. While the association between anaemia and poor prognosis, symptoms and hospitalization has been demonstrated consistently in various studies, a 'cause and effect' link has never been identified. Whilst it would seem an attractive concept to correct the anaemia, there is as yet no clear evidence that such a correction would lead to a better outcome, with most clinical trials having been small and nonrandomized in design. Thus, the heart failure specialist is well placed to coordinate investigations of anaemia with hospital colleagues, and to facilitate therapy with iron and erythropoietin if thought appropriate.

Renal failure

Renal failure is a common feature of patients with heart failure, being present in up to 50% of cases [33]. Numerous studies have shown consistently that renal impairment is associated with a poor outcome in heart failure [34], even when controlled for other risk factors [33]. There is some evidence to suggest that renal failure may even be a stronger predictor of clinical events than LV function [35]. In patients with mild renal insufficiency, ACE inhibitors and beta-blockers have been shown as safe [35, 36]. Not all renal failure in CHF is due to heart failure, however, and in this situation the heart failure specialist will normally coordinate with colleagues providing renal care. Indeed, in more advanced renal impairment a joint approach to management may well be required.

Atrial fibrillation/flutter

Congestive heart failure predisposes to atrial fibrillation (AF). Indeed, data obtained from the Framingham Study suggested that CHF was associated with a 4.5- to sixfold risk of AF in both men and women [39]. These two cardiac disorders are inextricably linked, with patients having one of these disorders being at substantially increased risk of developing the other. Atrial fibrillation is common in patients with LV systolic dysfunction, regardless of the underlying aetiology, and the prevalence of AF in patients with CHF ranges from 10 to 50%, depending on the severity of the CHF. Atrial fibrillation in CHF patients is also associated with increased mortality and morbidity [40]. The treatment of AF traditionally involves two objectives: (i) the prevention of thromboembolic complications; and (ii) rate or rhythm control.

The risk of thromboembolic stroke in older patients with AF is approximately 8% per year, and this is further increased by approximately 40% in the presence of CHF [41]. In general, adjusted-dose oral anticoagulation is highly effective for the prevention of both ischaemic and haemorrhagic strokes, with a risk reduction of about 60%; the absolute risk reduction is 3% a year in primary prevention and 8% a year in secondary prevention.

The treatment of AF often involves assessing the relative merits of rate control versus rhythm control. In a rate-control strategy, it is accepted that the patient will remain in AF and that all effort is directed towards rate control with single or combination medications, or even atrioventricular (AV) node ablation and PPM implantation if pharmacological agents are ineffective. In a rhythm-control strategy, efforts are directed towards the restoration and maintenance of sinus rhythm. It is assumed that the maintenance of sinus rhythm will improve the haemodynamics and so will be better in the long term. Whilst, in theory, it makes sense to maintain sinus rhythm, the medications used are potentially toxic. So, which is best - rate or rhythm control? Two major trials have confirmed that rate control is at least as effective as rhythm control [42, 43], while the National Institute for Health and Clinical Excellence (NICE) Guidelines provide specific advice about the treatment of AF.

For the treatment of refractory patients, AV node ablation with PPM implantation may be considered. This approach has been shown to be effective, improving symptom control and decreasing hospitalization [44].

Catheter-based ablation (as opposed to AV nodal ablation) for AF has shown much promise in the treatment of CHF. The restoration and maintenance of sinus rhythm by catheter ablation, without the use of drugs and without a need for PPM implantation in patients with CHF and AF, was shown to cause significant improvements in cardiac function, symptoms, exercise capacity and quality of life [44].

The treatment of atrial flutter is the same as for AF. However, atrial flutter is more amenable to ablation, and all patients should be referred for consideration of this procedure.

11.8 Multidisciplinary care (see also Chapter 13)

Congestive heart failure is a multifaceted problem that cannot be optimally managed by a single practitioner. Comprehensive disease-management programmes have been shown to improve the quality of CHF care in older patients [45], and the NICE guidelines have provided valuable insights and frameworks to specify a heart failure service for the management of chronic heart failure, although no one strategy is appropriate for all clinical settings. Nonetheless, the heart failure cardiologist and members of their team are integral to all successful care models; many programmes include specialized multidisciplinary heart failure clinics led by cardiologists or heart failure specialists, or conducted by nurses or nurse practitioners who can call on other health care professionals when necessary (see Figure 11.1). Heart failure specialists often see it as their responsibility to establish and develop a care programme that is specific to the local situation.

Nursing care

The role of the specialist nurse is discussed in detail in Chapter 10. These nurses potentially have a pivotal role in liaising between primary and secondary care, but for this to be effective the nurse must work closely with the heart failure specialist. This will ensure better communication between primary and secondary care with regards to individual patients, and also provide essential educational support for the nurse.

Palliative care issues (see Chapter 14)

The topic of the palliative care needs of patients with heart failure has been extensively aired in recent years [46–48]. During this time, it has become increasingly clear that the most appropriate health care professions to provide palliative support

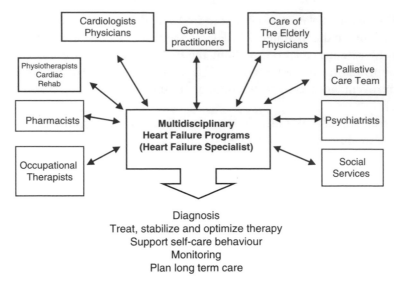

Figure 11.1   A multidisciplinary approach is required to deliver a high-quality heart failure service.

for these patients are those who manage their cardiological problems on a day-to-day basis, and not those who primarily work in palliative care. The heart failure specialist has an important role to play in establishing this support locally and in encouraging the involvement of colleagues.

Although patients complain about being poorly informed about the various aspects of their disease by their professional carers, heart failure specialists or members of their team are often the first to be able to discuss with patients the full significance and treatment options of their diagnosis. Having done this at the appropriate time, the details of the discussions should be relayed to the GP and others involved in the patient's care in order to minimize the risk of another common complaint from patients – that of receiving mixed messages.

Advanced heart failure is the point in the disease's natural history when the patient's symptoms become noticeably resistant to conventional medication. This identifies the need to introduce a palliative strategy for symptom control, for example an opiate regimen to relieve breathlessness. Although many doctors are unaware of (or reluctant to use) this treatment, heart failure specialists see many patients at this stage of the disease, either in clinic or during hospitalization. Hence, they should make a point of advising and encouraging the GP to trial the palliative care options for symptom control. Such an opportunity should also be taken to advise that the patient be included on the practice palliative care register.

Local treatment guidelines

The treatment of heart failure (see Chapter 6) is largely based on the outcome of randomized controlled clinical trials which are detailed, along with other aspects of patient management, in national and international guidelines. Despite this, the majority of patients still do not receive the optimum standard medication and other (non-pharmacological) components of a management programme. In this situation the heart failure specialist can, in collaboration with others, develop and maintain locally relevant management guidelines. In addition to providing advice about standard medications, it would for example highlight the criteria for recommending device therapy and surgery. This should – but does not always – ensure that all those involved in caring for heart failure patients in their locality are '. . .singing from the same hymn sheet'. This will in turn minimize any misunderstanding between health care professionals about the most appropriate treatment, and also avoid confusion in the minds of patients and their carers regarding their management.

Acknowledgement

Dr Pauriah was supported by a grant from the Translational Medicine Research Collaboration, and Dr Aaron Wong was supported by a grant from the British Heart Foundation. We are grateful to Andrew Rankine for his technical assistance in the preparation of this chapter.

References

1. Rutten, F.H., Grobbee, D.E. and Hoes, A.W. (2003) Differences between general practitioners and cardiologists in diagnosis and management of heart failure: a survey in every-day practice. *European Journal of Heart Failure*, **5** (3), 337–344.
2. Foody, J.M., Rathore, S.S., Wang, Y. *et al.* (2005) Physician specialty and mortality among elderly patients hospitalized with heart failure. *The American Journal of Medicine*, **118** (10), 1120–1125.
3. Roccaforte, R., Demers, C., Baldassarre, F. *et al.* (2005) Effectiveness of comprehensive disease management programmes in improving clinical outcomes in heart failure patients. A meta-analysis. *European Journal of Heart Failure*, **7** (7), 1133–1144.
4. Gray, A., Goodacre, S., Newby, D.E. *et al.* (2008) Noninvasive ventilation in acute cardiogenic pulmonary edema. *The New England Journal of Medicine*, **359** (2), 142–151.
5. Cintron, G., Bigas, C., Linares, E. *et al.* (1983) Nurse practitioner role in a chronic congestive heart failure clinic: in-hospital time, costs, and patient satisfaction. *Heart and Lung*, **12** (3), 237–240.

6. Kornowski, R., Zeeli, D., Averbuch, M. *et al.* (1995) Intensive home-care surveillance prevents hospitalization and improves morbidity rates among elderly patients with severe congestive heart failure. *American Heart Journal*, **129** (4), 762–766.

7. Lehtonen, L. and Poder, P. (2007) The utility of levosimendan in the treatment of heart failure. *Annals of Medicine*, **39** (1), 2–17.

8. Costanzo, M.R., Guglin, M.E., Saltzberg, M.T. *et al.* (2007) Ultrafiltration versus intravenous diuretics for patients hospitalized for acute decompensated heart failure. *Journal of the American College of Cardiology*, **49** (6), 675–683.

9. Yancy, C.W. (2007) Benefit-risk assessment of nesiritide in the treatment of acute decompensated heart failure. *Drug Safety*, **30** (9), 765–781.

10. deGoma, E.M., Vagelos, R.H., Fowler, M.B. and Ashley, E.A. (2006) Emerging therapies for the management of decompensated heart failure: from bench to bedside. *Journal of the American College of Cardiology*, **48** (12), 2397–2409.

11. Vallon, V., Miracle, C. and Thomson, S. (2008) Adenosine and kidney function: potential implications in patients with heart failure. *European Journal of Heart Failure*, **10** (2), 176–187.

12. Ali, F., Raufi, M.A., Washington, B. and Ghali, J.K. (2007) Conivaptan: a dual vasopressin receptor v1a/v2 antagonist [corrected]. *Cardiovascular Drug Reviews*, **25** (3), 261–279.

13. Gregoratos, G., Abrams, J., Epstein, A.E. *et al.* (2002) ACC/AHA/NASPE 2002 guideline update for implantation of cardiac pacemakers and antiarrhythmia devices: summary article: a report of the American College of Cardiology/American Heart Association Task Force on Practice Guidelines (ACC/AHA/NASPE Committee to Update the 1998 Pacemaker Guidelines). *Circulation*, **106** (16), 2145–2161.

14. Su, H., Lang, C., Noman, A. *et al.* (2007) Right ventricular pacing worsens endothelial function. *Journal of Cardiac Failure*, **13**, S126.

15. Bardy, G.H., Lee, K.L., Mark, D.B. *et al.* (2005) Amiodarone or an implantable cardioverter-defibrillator for congestive heart failure. *The New England Journal of Medicine*, **352** (3), 225–237.

16. Cleland, J.G., Daubert, J.C., Erdmann, E. *et al.* (2005) The effect of cardiac resynchronization on morbidity and mortality in heart failure. *The New England Journal of Medicine*, **352** (15), 1539–1549.

17. Delnoy, P.P., Ottervanger, J.P., Luttikhuis, H.O. *et al.* (2008) Clinical response of cardiac resynchronization therapy in the elderly. *American Heart Journal*, **155** (4), 746–751.

18. Phillips, H.R., O'Connor, C.M. and Rogers, J. (2007) Revascularization for heart failure. *American Heart Journal*, **153** (4 Suppl), 65–73.

19. LaCroix, A.Z., Guralnik, J.M., Curb, J.D. *et al.* (1990) Chest pain and coronary heart disease mortality among older men and women in three communities. *Circulation*, **81** (2), 437–446.

20. Batchelor, W.B., Anstrom, K.J., Muhlbaier, L.H. *et al.* (2000) Contemporary outcome trends in the elderly undergoing percutaneous coronary interventions: results in 7,472 octogenarians. National Cardiovascular Network Collaboration. *Journal of the American College of Cardiology*, **36** (3), 723–730.

21. Costa, J.R. Jr, Sousa, A., Moreira, A.C. *et al.* (2008) Drug-eluting stents in the elderly: long-term (>one year) clinical outcomes of octogenarians in the DESIRE (Drug-Eluting Stents In the REal world) registry. *The Journal of Invasive Cardiology*, **20** (8), 404–410.

22. Sukiennik, A., Krol, A., Jachalska, A. *et al.* (2007) Percutaneous coronary angioplasty in elderly patients: Assessment of in-hospital outcomes. *Cardiology Journal*, **14** (2), 143–154.

23. Guo, L., Mai, X., Deng, J. *et al.* (2008) Early percutaneous intervention improves survival in elderly patients with acute myocardial infarction complicated by cardiogenic shock. *Kardiologia Polska*, **66** (7), 722–726.

24. Alderman, E.L., Fisher, L.D., Litwin, P. *et al.* (1983) Results of coronary artery surgery in patients with poor left ventricular function (CASS). *Circulation*, **68** (4), 785–795.

25. Bouma, B.J., van der Meulen, J.H., van den Brink, R.B. *et al.* (2001) Variability in treatment advice for elderly patients with aortic stenosis: a nationwide survey in The Netherlands. *Heart (British Cardiac Society)*, **85** (2), 196–201.

26. Iung, B., Baron, G., Butchart, E.G. *et al.* (2003) A prospective survey of patients with valvular heart disease in Europe: The Euro Heart Survey on Valvular Heart Disease. *European Heart Journal*, **24** (13), 1231–1243.

27. Monin, J.L., Quere, J.P., Monchi, M. *et al.* (2003) Low-gradient aortic stenosis: operative risk stratification and predictors for long-term outcome: a multicenter study using dobutamine stress hemodynamics. *Circulation*, **108** (3), 319–324.

28. Wong, J.B., Salem, D.N. and Pauker, S.G. (1993) You're never too old. *The New England Journal of Medicine*, **328** (13), 971–975.

29. Enriquez-Sarano, M., Tajik, A.J., Schaff, H.V. *et al.* (1994) Echocardiographic prediction of survival after surgical correction of organic mitral regurgitation. *Circulation*, **90** (2), 830–837.

30. Bonow, R.O., Carabello, B.A., Chatterjee, K. *et al.* (2006) ACC/AHA 2006 guidelines for the management of patients with valvular heart disease: a report of the American College of Cardiology/American Heart Association Task Force on Practice Guidelines (writing Committee to Revise the 1998 guidelines for the management of patients with valvular heart disease) developed in collaboration with the Society of Cardiovascular Anesthesiologists endorsed by the Society for Cardiovascular Angiography and Interventions and the Society of Thoracic Surgeons. *Journal of the American College of Cardiology*, **48** (3), e1–148.

31. van der Meer, P., Voors, A.A., Lipsic, E. *et al.* (2004) Erythropoietin in cardiovascular diseases. *European Heart Journal*, **25** (4), 285–291.

32. Horwich, T.B., Fonarow, G.C., Hamilton, M.A. *et al.* (2002) Anemia is associated with worse symptoms, greater impairment in functional capacity and a significant increase in mortality in patients with advanced heart failure. *Journal of the American College of Cardiology*, **39** (11), 1780–1786.

33. McAlister, F.A., Ezekowitz, J., Tonelli, M. and Armstrong, P.W. (2004) Renal insufficiency and heart failure: prognostic and therapeutic implications from a prospective cohort study. *Circulation*, **109** (8), 1004–1009.

34. McClellan, W.M., Flanders, W.D., Langston, R.D. *et al.* (2002) Anemia and renal insufficiency are independent risk factors for death among patients with congestive heart failure admitted to community hospitals: a population-based study. *Journal of the American Society of Nephrology*, **13** (7), 1928–1936.

35. Hillege, H.L., Girbes, A.R., de Kam, P.J. *et al.* (2000) Renal function, neurohormonal activation, and survival in patients with chronic heart failure. *Circulation*, **102** (2), 203–210.

36. Mann, J.F., Gerstein, H.C., Pogue, J. *et al.* (2001) Renal insufficiency as a predictor of cardiovascular outcomes and the impact of ramipril: the HOPE randomized trial. *Annals of Internal Medicine*, **134** (8), 629–636.

37. Erdmann, E., Lechat, P., Verkenne, P. and Wiemann, H. (2001) Results from post-hoc analyses of the CIBIS II trial: effect of bisoprolol in high-risk patient groups with chronic heart failure. *European Journal of Heart Failure*, **3** (4), 469–479.

38. de Groote, P., Isnard, R., Assyag, P. *et al.* (2007) Is the gap between guidelines and clinical practice in heart failure treatment being filled? Insights from the IMPACT RECO survey. *European Journal of Heart Failure*, **9** (12), 1205–1211.

39. Kannel, W.B., Wolf, P.A., Benjamin, E.J. and Levy, D. (1998) Prevalence, incidence, prognosis, and predisposing conditions for atrial fibrillation: population-based estimates. *The American Journal of Cardiology*, **82** (8A), 2N–9N.

40. Wang, T.J., Larson, M.G., Levy, D. *et al.* (2003) Temporal relations of atrial fibrillation and congestive heart failure and their joint influence on mortality: the Framingham Heart Study. *Circulation*, **107** (23), 2920–2925.

41. Fuster, V., Ryden, L.E., Cannom, D.S. *et al.* (2006) ACC/AHA/ESC 2006 Guidelines for the Management of Patients with Atrial Fibrillation: a report of the American College of Cardiology/American Heart Association Task Force on Practice Guidelines and the European Society of Cardiology Committee for Practice Guidelines (Writing Committee to Revise the 2001 Guidelines for the Management of Patients With Atrial Fibrillation): developed in collaboration with the European Heart Rhythm Association and the Heart Rhythm Society. *Circulation*, **114** (7), e257–354.

42. Wyse, D.G., Waldo, A.L., DiMarco, J.P. *et al.* (2002) A comparison of rate control and rhythm control in patients with atrial fibrillation. *The New England Journal of Medicine*, **347** (23), 1825–1833.

43. Van Gelder, I.C., Hagens, V.E., Bosker, H.A. *et al.* (2002) A comparison of rate control and rhythm control in patients with recurrent persistent atrial fibrillation. *The New England Journal of Medicine*, **347** (23), 1834–1840.

44. Hsu, L.F., Jais, P., Sanders, P. *et al.* (2004) Catheter ablation for atrial fibrillation in congestive heart failure. *The New England Journal of Medicine*, **351** (23), 2373–2383.

45. Gonseth, J., Guallar-Castillon, P., Banegas, J.R. and Rodriguez-Artalejo, F. (2004) The effectiveness of disease management programmes in reducing hospital re-admission in older patients with heart failure: a systematic review and meta-analysis of published reports. *European Heart Journal*, **25** (18), 1570–1595.

46. Stewart, S., MacIntyre, K., Hole, D.J. *et al.* (2001) More 'malignant' than cancer? Five-year survival following a first admission for heart failure. *European Journal of Heart Failure*, **3** (3), 315–322.
47. Remme, W.J., McMurray, J.J., Rauch, B. *et al.* (2005) Public awareness of heart failure in Europe: first results from SHAPE. *European Heart Journal*, **26** (22), 2413–2421.
48. Stromberg, A. and Jaarsma, T. (2008) Thoughts about death and perceived health status in elderly patients with heart failure. *European Journal of Heart Failure*, **10** (6), 608–613.
49. Lang, C.C. and Mancini, D.M. (2007) Non-cardiac comorbidities in chronic heart failure. *Heart (British Cardiac Society)*, **93** (6), 665–671.

12

Hospitalization

Andrew Hannah

Department of Cardiology, Aberdeen Royal Infirmary, Aberdeen

Key messages

- Heart failure is the leading cause of hospitalization in older patients.

- Approximately 50% of these episodes of hospitalization are directly related to the heart; an acute coronary syndrome, atrial fibrillation, hypertension or progression of known left ventricular impairment.

- Most of the remaining admissions are the result of problems associated with medications or a comorbidity.

- At least a half of all hospitalizations could be prevented by relatively simple measures.

12.1 The epidemiology of hospitalization

At any one time, heart failure affects an estimated 800 000 people in the United Kingdom, with the incidence and prevalence rising markedly in older people. To place this in context, an estimated 1 in 35 people aged between 65 and 74 years will have heart failure, compared to 1 in 15 aged 75 to 84 years, and 1 in 7 aged 85 years and above [1]. The condition is characterized by a high mortality and a high morbidity; a major reason for such high morbidity is hospitalization that is often recurrent and can often be prolonged [2].

A Practical Guide to Heart Failure in Older People, Edited by C Ward and M D Witham
© 2009 John Wiley & Sons, Ltd

The UK Department of Health statistics from 2000/2001 suggest that there were approximately 74 500 hospital admissions in England and 13 500 in Scotland with a principal diagnosis of heart failure. These numbers account for approximately 2% of all hospital admissions, and up to 2% of total 'bed-days'. Furthermore, an additional 1.5% of total hospital admissions and 1.9% of total bed-days pertained to patients admitted with a secondary diagnosis of heart failure [3]. A very similar level of heart failure hospitalizations is seen across Western and Northern Europe [4].

Because, as noted above, heart failure is a disease of older people, the majority of hospitalized patients inevitably also tend to be older. The average age of patients admitted with cardiac decompensation is 75–78 years and appears to be rising, particularly among males. Although the prognosis remains poor for such patients there are trends towards better survival despite the increasing age [5, 6].

The economic burden of heart failure management in the UK is enormous, as it consumes approximately 1–2% of the country's total health care costs, with up to 75% of this pertaining to the cost of hospitalization. The reason for this is twofold: Firstly, hospitalization of heart failure patients is common; and second the average length of stay is approximately 14 days.

One of the major focuses of heart failure management must therefore be to reduce the number and length of hospital admissions; any successful strategy is likely to be cost-effective.

12.2 The aetiology of heart failure in hospitalized patients

The aetiology of heart failure in hospitalized patients is very similar to that in the wider heart failure population, in that a history of ischaemic heart disease and/or hypertension is present in approximately two-thirds of patients: with some 35% have significant valvular disease. Some comorbidities – notably diabetes, renal failure, atrial fibrillation and hypertension – play an important aetiological role (see Chapters 4 and 8).

The underlying cardiac pathophysiology is also similar to that of heart failure in general. Significant left ventricular (LV) systolic dysfunction is present in 45–65% of cases, which is perhaps slightly more frequent than in an outpatient population. Heart failure with preserved LV systolic function (HF-PSF) is the diagnosis in the majority of remaining patients; this was present in just over one-third of patients in the EuroHeart Failure Survey II, more so in those presenting with acute *de novo* heart failure than in decompensated chronic heart failure (see below). However, in the ADHERE registry, and some other smaller studies, the prevalence of HF-PSF was over 50%. This group of patients tends to be older, a higher percentage is female and there is a high prevalence of hypertension and diabetes, but they are less likely to have a history of myocardial infarction or ischaemic heart disease [7].

Valvular dysfunction appears to be more common among hospitalized patients. For example, in the EuroHeart Failure Survey II [8] over 40% of patients had moderate or severe valvular dysfunction, and this rose to over 50% in acute decompensated heart failure. Moreover, 80% of these patients had evidence of mitral regurgitation (MR), in approximately half of whom it was moderate or severe. In a large majority, the MR regurgitation was functional rather than valvular (see Chapter 4). Other valve abnormalities such as functional tricuspid regurgitation were also prevalent, but some cases were due to primary valvular disease, notably aortic stenosis.

12.3 Classification and diagnosis of acute heart failure (AHF)

Classification

Patients who are admitted primarily because of heart failure (see below) have been subdivided into those with acute *de novo* heart failure (*de novo* AHF) and those with acute decompensated heart failure (ADHF) [8]. There are some major differences between these groups with respect to precipitating factors and, as discussed later, the concept of 'preventable causes' is more relevant to the acutely decompensated group.

- The term *de novo* AHF is applied to those cases without a prior diagnosis of, or admission with, heart failure.

- ADHF refers to patients with a pre-existing diagnosis of heart failure or with known asymptomatic LV systolic dysfunction.

In both groups the onset of symptoms may be sudden and life threatening.

Acute heart failure has also been classified according to the dominant clinical signs as suggested by the European Society of Cardiology [9]: Acute decompensated HF, hypertensive heart failure, pulmonary oedema, cardiogenic shock, right-heart failure and 'high-output' heart failure. There is inevitably some overlap between these groups, but the classification highlights the fact that the focus of management varies between the groups, as is evident from the data in Table 12.1.

Diagnosis

The specific difficulties of diagnosing heart failure in older people are discussed in Chapter 5 and in Refs [10–12]. In the context of hospitalized patients it should be noted that those with previously diagnosed and treated chronic heart failure often

Table 12.1 The classification of acute heart failure. Based on data from Ref. [9].

Type of acute heart failure	Clinical features
Acute decompensated HF	Clinical features of HF which do not fulfil criteria for other types
Hypertensive heart failure	Signs of HF accompanied by marked hypertension (typically >180/100 mmHg)
Pulmonary oedema	Chest crepitations, orthopnoea, with respiratory distress and marked hypoxia on air (oedema confirmed on chest X-ray)
Cardiogenic shock	Evidence of tissue hypoperfusion in context of adequate preload. Hypotension (usually systolic BP <90 mmHg) with accompanying oliguria and pulse rate >60 bpm
Right-heart failure	Typically a low-output state with elevation of jugular venous pressure, exclusively peripheral oedema and often hypotension
High-output cardiac failure	By definition, preserved systolic function, usually marked tachycardia, sometimes warm peripheries and often due to noncardiac cause, for example anaemia, thyrotoxicoxis or iatrogenic fluid overload

have marked peripheral oedema, and although pulmonary oedema may also occur it is usually less marked or absent. By contrast, in *de novo* AHF – particularly in the context of an acute coronary syndrome or the recent onset of an arrhythmia (see below) – there is often more marked pulmonary oedema, with little or no peripheral oedema.

The investigation of heart failure, including the place of echocardiography and other imaging techniques (see Table 12.2), is discussed in Chapters 5 and 11.

Table 12.2 Summary of routine laboratory investigations of older patients hospitalized because of *de novo* or decompensated heart failure.

Urea and electrolytes	Always
Full blood count	Always
Liver function tests	Always
Glucose	Always
Thyroid function	Always
CRP[a]/ESR[b]	Always – to look for infection as a precipitant
Troponin	Usually (always in acute *de novo* HF)
BNP/NT-pro-BNP[c]	Usually/if available/if diagnostic doubt

[a]CRP = C-reactive protein.
[b]ESR = Erythrocyte sedimentation rate.
[c]BNP = B-type natriuretic protein.

12.4 Causes and precipitants of hospitalization

As older heart failure patients usually have multiple comorbidities and take numerous medications, frequently in less than ideal social circumstances, it is often difficult to identify one specific cause for their hospitalization. Consequently, having identified one likely explanation, other possible contributing factors should always be sought.

A precipitating or causative factor can be identified in 75–85% of patients hospitalized because of decompensation of known chronic heart failure [13, 14]. In many cases these hospitalizations could be prevented, or at least the severity of the symptoms modified [14–16]. A list of the most common precipitating factors is provided in Table 12.3, although there are marked variations in their reported frequency. Some of this variation relates to the population of patients studied, perhaps the health care setting, or to methodological issues relating to definitions of conditions, and in particular how actively any evidence of 'noncompliance' was sought. Even when an unequivocal precipitating factor may have been identified, there is often a degree of subjectivity involved in the process.

Cardiovascular causes

If sufficiently severe, almost any acute cardiac event or structural abnormality may precipitate acute heart failure, even in patients with relatively normal premorbid

Table 12.3 Common causes and precipitants of hospitalization in older patients with heart failure.

Cardiovascular
    Myocardial ischaemia/infarction
    Arrhythmias
    Uncontrolled hypertension
    Valvular dysfunction

Medication/lifestyle
    Lack of adherence to medications
    Withdrawal of medications
    Lack of adherence to dietary advice
    Harmful medications
    Unaccustomed physical effort
    Emotional stress

Comorbidities
    Anaemia
    Infections
    Worsening renal function

cardiac function. However, in patients with established chronic heart failure, relatively minor events have a high probability of precipitating decompensation, and this becomes more likely in those who are old and frail.

Despite the frequent difficulty of identifying the primary cause for hospitalization in a patient with heart failure, there is a consensus that heart failure *per se* is the likeliest explanation in the majority of cases.

Although heart failure is the most common cause of hospital admission in patients aged over 65, it is only in recent years that we have begun to accrue high-quality data based on large numbers of such patients in registries such as the ADHERE registry [17, 18] and the EuroHeart surveys [8] in the US and Europe, respectively. Such data are providing some insight into 'the real world' management and outcomes of hospitalized heart failure patients; perhaps more importantly, they also provide information about precipitating factors.

Acute coronary syndromes

Acute coronary syndrome (ACS) patients with ST elevation myocardial infarction (STEMI) and non-ST elevation myocardial infarction (NSTEMI) aged between 70 and 80 years have a twofold increased risk of death, cardiogenic shock and heart failure compared to younger patients, while patients aged >80 years have a five- to sixfold increase in the risk of early and late mortality (see Chapter 3).

A striking feature of acute *de novo* HF is the frequency with which an ACS is the precipitating/causative factor. Approximately 40% of patients with acute heart failure have an ACS, there being an approximately equal split between STEMI and non-STEMI, with a minority having troponin-negative unstable angina [8].

Although less common than in *de novo* heart failure, an ACS was also responsible for over 20% of hospitalizations in patients with prior heart failure in the EuroHeart Failure Survey II [8]. However, in contrast to *de novo* HF the form that the ACS took was different, with unstable angina being most common, followed by NSTEMI, and only 6% due to STEMI.

Arrhythmias

Arrhythmias account for between 15 and 30% of hospital admissions, and are probably the most common cardiac precipitant identified if the *de novo* and acute decompensated groups are combined. Ventricular arrhythmias are clearly very important in terms of predicting a short- and longer-term prognosis, although in numerical terms they account for very few heart failure-related hospitalizations. More commonly, it is a supraventricular arrhythmia – in particular atrial fibrillation

(AF) or atrial flutter – that causes decompensation. In the Euro Heart Failure Survey II [8], 32% of patients were felt to have decompensated because of an arrhythmia, and 46% of the ADCHF group had a prior diagnosis of one or the other of these arrhythmias. This is not surprising as it is well known that AF becomes more common with increasing severity of heart failure, with worsening NYHA functional class, and in older people.

Uncontrolled hypertension

Uncontrolled hypertension is thought to be a precipitating factor in 5–15% of heart failure admissions, although the reported frequency is very variable. A history of hypertension is found in up to two-thirds of patients in most studies, with the variance most likely being due mainly to the subjective nature of deciding the precipitant and the lack of any clear definition of hypertension in the context of acute HF. The European Society of Cardiology has suggested a definition of hypertensive heart failure as a blood pressure >180/100 mmHg with clinical signs of heart failure.

This mode of presentation is more likely in older female patients and in those with preserved LV systolic function (HF-PSF). It is noteworthy that these patients have the lowest in-hospital mortality rate of any of the heart failure subgroups, as well as having on average shorter duration of stay, reduced readmission for HF and a better medium-term prognosis. This is perhaps because the control of this causative factor can be relatively straightforward with appropriate combination drug therapies.

Noncardiac causes

Nonadherence to treatment is not unique to heart failure therapies, and seems to be increasingly prevalent in older populations and when polypharmacy exists. It is no surprise then that the typical older heart failure patient who is frequently taking six or more cardiac medications, often in addition to multiple noncardiac medications, will be prone to poor adherence. This is often based on poor patient education, both in terms of what tablets they should be taking and when, but also importantly why (see below).

Patient nonadherence with prescribed heart failure medications has been implicated in precipitating hospital admission in between 20 and 60% of cases [13, 16, 19, 20]. Pharmacological therapy is the cornerstone of modern heart failure management, but with these advances comes an increasing complexity of the drug regime. Furthermore, there may be unpleasant effects or side effects with a number of cardiac medicines: the diuresis related to diuretic therapy may cause social inconvenience and incontinence in older people; the benefits of an ACE inhibitor may not be apparent to the patient because of the delay in symptomatic improvement; and beta-blockers may initially cause worsening dyspnoea and be blamed for fatigue.

Other medication-related causes

The taking of harmful medications, such as non-steroidal anti-inflammatory drugs (NSAIDs) or the prescription of steroids, rate-limiting calcium channel blockers or doxazosin, contribute to some hospitalizations. In particular, there is evidence that NSAID use increases the risk of first hospitalizations for heart failure in patients with a pre-existing diagnosis of stable heart failure, and also for patients with no pre-existing diagnosis of heart failure [21] (see also Chapter 6).

The withdrawal of heart failure medications, such as beta-blockers or ACE inhibitors, may cause decompensation and hospitalization. Often, these changes are made for inappropriate reasons such as mild deterioration in renal function, cough (when an angiotensin-receptor blocker should be substituted for an ACE inhibitor), asymptomatic hypotension or fatigue.

Dietary factors such as a high salt or water intake are felt to play a role in approximately 5% of cases, with a similar number due to 'excessive' or more likely unaccustomed physical exertion or emotional stress.

Comorbidities

Other than medication and lifestyle issues, the principal noncardiac causes are related to comorbidities, notably infections, anaemia and renal dysfunction.

In some studies, infections are the single most common precipitating factor, more frequent than ACS or an arrhythmia. Clearly, with any infection if sufficiently severe – or if the control of heart failure is precarious – cardiac decompensation may occur. However, respiratory tract infections comprise the vast majority of the identified infections, and this probably reflects the high prevalence of chronic obstructive pulmonary disease (COPD) in heart failure, and the associated destabilizing effect of hypoxia.

Anaemia is frequently present in patients with advanced heart failure, with approximately 15% of patients who are hospitalized being anaemic [22, 23]. Occasionally, anaemia is felt to be the dominant precipitating factor, although epidemiologically there is little detailed information on what the cause and severity of the anaemia is under these circumstances. Certainly, anaemia if sufficiently severe will cause increased dyspnoea and sometimes frank decompensation. The aetiology of anaemia in these circumstances is heterogeneous and may be due to vitamin deficiencies, chronic blood loss, megaloblastosis, chronic renal failure or other chronic diseases, including HF itself.

Renal dysfunction is common in, and inter-related to, heart failure; it is a common cause or contributing factor to hospitalization (see Chapters 6 and 8).

12.5 Treatment of acute heart failure

Heart failure specialists have expertise in the detailed management of heart failure (see Chapter 11), although in the UK only a minority of patients hospitalized because of heart failure are under their care – or that of other cardiologists. Most patients are treated by general and care-of-the-elderly physicians, with specialist advice available from a cardiologist if necessary.

The principles of treatment, particularly the appropriate use of diuretics, as outlined here, are based on Refs [9, 17, 18].

There are four phases to the medical management of a patient admitted with acute heart failure:

- Phase 1: Establish haemodynamic stability and adequate oxygenation.

- Phase 2: Achieve euvolaemia and initiate appropriate long-term drug therapy.

- Phase 3: Optimize long-term drug therapy and patient education and establish mechanisms to ensure optimal and comprehensive post-discharge heart failure management.

- Phase 4: Ensure that a comprehensive review of other problems, comorbid diseases, physical and psychosocial function takes place, and put in place detailed plans for discharge and follow-up.

Phase 1: establish haemodynamic stability and adequate oxygenation

The details of how this is achieved depends on:

- The underlying cause of the acute HF; for example, management is very different if the cause is an ACS as opposed to atrial fibrillation.

- The initial blood pressure.

- The degree of respiratory distress/hypoxia.

- Whether the patient is in established or impending cardiogenic shock (see Figure 12.1).

Phase 2: achieving euvolaemia

After an initial stabilization, ongoing management is next directed at achieving euvolaemia. This invariably requires the use of intravenous loop diuretics in adequate doses, often in combination with other (oral) diuretics with different

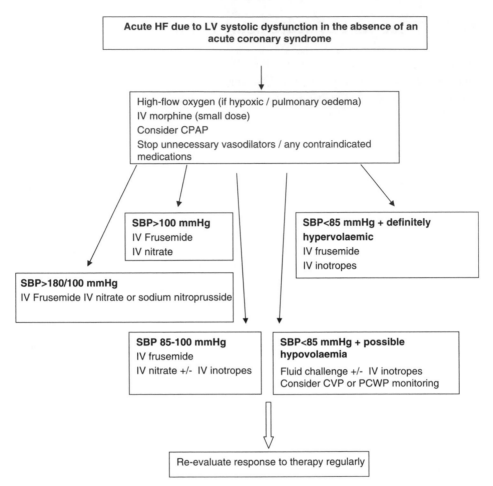

Figure 12.1 Algorithm summarizing the initial medical management of acute heart failure.

sites and modes of action within the kidney. The principles and use of diuretics are summarized in Tables 12.4 and 12.5.

Phase 3: optimizing heart failure therapies

Often, patients hospitalized with heart failure (especially *de novo* cases) will not be receiving any appropriate therapies; moreover, even when a relevant treatment is documented it may be suboptimal, both in terms of dosage and drug type. The average 7–14 days of in-hospital stay is therefore an excellent opportunity to optimize drug therapies, to educate the patient and his/her relatives, as well as to set out an ongoing management strategy for the future.

Table 12.4 Managing diuretic resistance.

Ensure IV administration of furosemide, preceded by bolus
Increase furosemide dose (especially in chronic kidney disease)
Continuous infusion rather than high-dose bolus
Combination diuretics
   Loop/bendroflumethiazide (not useful if significant renal impairment)
   Loop/spironolactone
   Loop/metolazone (best combination for renal failure.)
   Ensure adequate fluid restriction
Ensure adequate blood pressure
   if oliguric reduce ACE inhibitor and/or add inotropes
Combine aggressive diuretic therapy with low-dose inotropes (if BP <100 mmHg)
Consider ultrafiltration or haemodialysis

Phase 4: comprehensive review

Older patients with heart failure almost always suffer from a wide range of impairments and comorbid diseases. Indeed, it is worth remembering that such patients will often be admitted to hospital for reasons other than decompensation of their heart failure. Each hospital admission is therefore an opportunity to ensure that comprehensive assessment by the whole multidisciplinary team takes place. It is not uncommon, having optimized the management of heart failure, to discover that delirium, falls or poorly controlled diabetes stand in the way of a successful discharge or the ability to manage at home in the longer term.

As soon as euvolaemia is in sight, the next phase of assessment should begin. A review of other active diseases, cognition, psychological status, assessment by physiotherapy and occupational therapy, a review of current home care and current nursing needs are all required.

Timely decisions can then be taken regarding the need for rehabilitation and how much support will be needed in the community, thus allowing accurate discharge planning. The input of a geriatrician is usually invaluable at this stage.

Many early post-discharge readmissions are the result of patients being allowed home without optimum stabilization of their condition or of inadequate forward planning for their future care.

Table 12.5 Common pitfalls in diuretic use.

Using oral rather than IV administration
Inadequate dose (especially if renal failure present: higher dose required)
Failure to prescribe if hypotension present
Premature change to oral loop diuretic
Inadequate fluid balance monitoring

12.6   Management of the common cardiac causes of hospitalization for heart failure (see also Chapter 11)

Acute coronary syndromes in older patients

Despite the poor prognosis of ACS resulting in heart failure in older patients (see above), relatively few older patients undergo reperfusion (in the very old this is often <40%). The extent of prescription of evidence-based drug therapies in older ACS patients, particular of beta-blockers, statins and clopidogrel, is also lower than in younger patients.

An early invasive strategy for the management of NSTEMI offers improvement in mortality and morbidity for some patient groups. As an example, the TACTICS study suggested that a much greater benefit was seen in the older age groups than the young. This undoubtedly comes at the cost of increased bleeding and other complications [24, 25], although these problems can be minimized by attention to details such as a reduction in the dose of low-molecular-weight heparin in those with renal impairment, and the use of bivalirudin and radial vascular access for percutaneous coronary intervention. Even then, however, in the very old the risks probably outweigh the benefit.

Cardiogenic shock is the most extreme clinical presentation of acute heart failure, including those cases resulting from an ACS, and carries a dire prognosis in older patients. The routine use of an invasive strategy to address this appears, on current evidence, to offer no benefit to the over-75s, but should be considered in selected cases [26, 27].

Atrial fibrillation

Atrial fibrillation is present in up to 40% of patients hospitalized with HF. The only indication for immediate electrical cardioversion is the presence of haemodynamic instability, which usually occurs in the context of new-onset AF with a rapid ventricular rate (see Chapter 3). More commonly, the onset of AF results in a more insidious decompensation of heart failure. In all other cases a decision must be taken on whether to use a strategy of 'rate' or 'rhythm control', which depends on a number of factors [28] (see Chapters 6 and 11). There is however, little to choose between these strategies for most patients.

Hypertension

Despite the importance of hypertension as a cause of heart failure and as a precipitant of ADHF, older hypertensive patients tend to be under-treated or not treated at all.

There is, however, strong evidence that good hypertension control reduces heart failure episodes, and therefore in turn hospital admissions (by up to 50%), as well as a reduction in strokes, renal failure and perhaps dementia [29]. These worthwhile morbidity benefits may be far more important to older patients than a mortality benefit.

The treatment of hypertension in heart failure, with or without LV systolic dysfunction (LVSD), is the same as for non- heart failure patients, except that diltiazem, verapamil and nifedipine (and related nondihydropyridines) should be avoided in those with LVSD.

12.7 Outcomes in patients hospitalized for heart failure

Hospitalization as a result of heart failure is a serious event. Overall, there is a 6–9% risk of death during the index admission, whether the presentation is for '*de novo*' heart failure or ADHF. The presenting clinical features may, however, be important predictors of outcome. At the worst end of the spectrum, cardiogenic shock has an in-hospital mortality of 40–60%, whereas for decompensated hypertensive heart failure the in-hospital mortality is less than 2% [8].

Following discharge, patients remain at high risk; the mortality is approximately 10% during the first 1–3 months, and up to 30% by one year. A few studies have examined the longer-term prognosis and suggested mortalities of up to 60–75% by five years [30]. These figures may be considered to apply to older patients as the mean age of hospitalized patients is approximately 75 years. However, mortality rates continue to rise steeply with age and the prognosis for the 'very old' is >50% at one year [31].

Admission to hospital is also a strong predictor of future morbidity, frequently in the form of repeat hospitalizations [32, 33]. A number of registries and retrospective studies have suggested that the readmission rate is approximately 30% in the 3–6-month period following the index admission [7]. The pattern of readmissions appears to be 'front-loaded' – that is, the highest readmission rates tend to be in the first one to two months post discharge and diminish over the next 10–12 weeks. Clearly, not all readmissions are cardiac-related, and indeed some registries suggest that only about 25–50% are due to heart failure. Nevertheless, this remarkably high readmission rate must be considered a focus for 'interventions'.

Perhaps not surprisingly the prognosis of patients with repeated heart failure-related hospitalizations becomes progressively worse [34]. This seems to be true in the younger heart failure patient, as well as in those who are older. Conversely, although readmissions for noncardiac reasons are common in heart failure patients, these do not seem to predict higher mortality rates in the same way that repeat admissions for heart failure do. This would imply that readmissions for heart failure are not prognostically powerful simply as a marker of frailty, but more specifically indicate progression of the heart failure, a failure of treatment (or inadequate treatment), or both.

12.8   Strategies to reduce admissions and readmissions in patients with heart failure

Optimization of pharmacological therapies

In addition to improving mortality, drugs such as ACE inhibitors, beta-blockers and angiotensin- and aldosterone-receptor blockers have been shown to reduce the risk of heart failure-related hospitalization. This is true both in mild and advanced heart failure, including those who may have had multiple admissions. In order to reap the maximum benefits, these agents should therefore be titrated to full recommended therapeutic doses, or maximum tolerated dosage, acknowledging that this will be labour-intensive and may take several months to achieve.

The role of the heart failure specialist nurse

The term disease management programme (DMP) refers to a multidisciplinary team approach for the management of heart failure. In turn, the role of the heart failure specialist nurse (HFSN) appears to be a key element to all successful DMPs (see Chapters 10 and 13).

The group of heart failure patients who seem to have most to gain from such input are those who have been admitted with decompensated heart failure due to LVSD, especially if they have advanced heart failure – that is, those with severe symptoms despite a three-month treatment with optimum tolerated medication. It is this group who are at highest risk of (re-)admissions. Furthermore, the fact that noncompliance with prescribed medications is such a common cause of hospitalization may also indicate that they are the ideal group to target with intensive specialist nurse input.

Many HFSN programmes thus target patients during a hospital admission, or make contact at the time of discharge. Integration of the HFSN into the process of discharge planning is therefore vital; the HFSN must be contacted early enough during the course of a hospitalization to be able to have input into the discharge planning process, and to be able to make contact with the patient before discharge, to start the process of patient education, and to ensure that patients and carers understand what the medications are for, how to self-monitor, and who to contact if they feel unwell. (A fuller discussion of these issues is provided in Chapter 10.)

Preemptive monitoring

Much of the self-monitoring that patients are taught to undertake, for example weighing themselves at home and checking for ankle oedema, is done with a view to identifying decompensation at an early stage and thus avoiding hospital admission. Such information is demonstrably helpful in some cases, and again, HFSNs are ideally placed to provide the necessary early intervention when increased weight or ankle oedema appears.

Unfortunately, such monitoring is relatively crude, tends to detect problems relatively late, and cannot be done successfully by all older heart failure patients, notably those with cognitive impairment and/or a poor social support network. Ideally, the monitoring of fluid balance should be carried out electronically, and intrathoracic impedance monitoring offers the prospect of doing this. When a patient with heart failure decompensates, fluid retention results in both intravascular and extravascular volume expansion, and often also pulmonary oedema. These fluid changes lead to a decreased thoracic impedance, as the higher water content of tissues increases their electrical conduction [40]. Some pacemakers and implantable cardioverter defibrillators are able to measure intrathoracic impedance continuously, and some preliminary studies are beginning to investigate the practical merits of this with the prospect of pre-empting overt symptomatic deterioration.

References

1. Peterson, S., Rayner, M. and Wolstenholme, J. (2002) *Coronary Heart Disease Statistics: Heart Failure Supplement*. British Heart Foundation, London.
2. Bundkirchen, A. and Schwinger, R.H.G. (2004) Epidemiology and economic burden of chronic heart failure. *European Heart Journal*, **6** (Suppl D), D57–60.
3. British Heart Foundation: www.heartstats.org.
4. Cleland, J.G.F., Swedberg, K., Follath, F. *et al.* (2003) The EuroHeart Failure survey programme - a survey on the quality of care among patients with heart failure in Europe. Part 1. *European Heart Journal*, **24**, 442–463.
5. Blackledge, H.M., Tomlinson, J. and Squire, I.B. (2003) Prognosis for patients newly admitted to hospital with heart failure: survival trends in 12 220 index admissions in Leicestershire 1993–2001. *Heart*, **89**, 615–620.
6. Stewart, S., MacIntyre, K., Capewell, S. and McMurray, J.J.V. (2003) Heart failure and the aging population: an increasing burden in the 21st century? *Heart*, **89**, 49–53.
7. Fonarow, G.C., Stough, W.G., Abraham, W.T., Albert, N.M. *et al.* (2007) Characteristics, treatments and outcomes of patients with preserved systolic function hospitalised for heart failure: a report from the OPTIMIZE-HF registry. *Journal of the American College of Cardiology*, **50**, 768–777.

8. Niemenin, M.S., Brutsaert, D., Dickstein, K. *et al.* (2006) EuroHeart Failure Survey II (EHFS II): a survey on hospitalised acute heart failure patients: description of population. *European Heart Journal*, **27**, 2725–2736.

9. Task Force on Acute Heart Failure of the European Society of Cardiology (2005) Guidelines on the diagnosis and treatment of acute heart failure.

10. Wheeldon, N.M., MacDonald, T.M., Flucker, C.J., McKendrick, A.D. *et al.* (1993) Echocardiography in chronic heart failure in the community. *Quarterly Journal of Medicine*, **86**, 17–23.

11. Owen, A. and Cox, S. (2001) Diagnosis of heart failure in elderly patients in primary care. *European Journal of Heart Failure*, **3**, 79–81.

12. Mulrow, C.D., Lucey, C.R. and Famett, L.E. (1993) Discriminating causes of dyspnoea through clinical examination. *Journal of General Internal Medicine*, **8**, 383–392.

13. Formiga, F., Chivite, D., Manito, N., Casas, S. *et al.* (2007) Hospitalisation due to acute heart failure. Role of precipitating factors. *International Journal of Cardiology*, **120**, 237–241.

14. Michalsen, A., Konig, G. and Thimme, W. (1998) Preventable causative factors leading to hospital admission with decompensated heart failure. *Heart*, **80**, 437–441.

15. Opasich, C., Febo, O., Riccardi, G. *et al.* (1996) Concomitant factors of decompensation in chronic heart failure. *American Journal of Cardiology*, **78**, 354–357.

16. Ghali, J.K., Kadakia, S., Cooper, R. and Ferlinz, J. (1988) Precipitating factors leading to decompensation of heart failure: traits among urban blacks. *Archives of Internal Medicine*, **148**, 2013–2016.

17. Gheorghiade, M. and Filippatos, G. (2005) Reassessing treatment of acute heart failure syndromes: the ADHERE Registry. *European Heart Journal Supplements*, **7** (Suppl B), B13–19.

18. Fonarow, G.C. (2003) The acute decompensated heart failure national registry (ADHERE): opportunities to improve care of patients hospitalised with acute decompensated heart failure. *Reviews in Cardiovascular Medicine*, **4** (Suppl 7), S21–S30.

19. Tsuyuki, R.T., McKelvie, R.S., Arnold, J.M., Avezum, A. *et al.* (2001) Acute precipitants of congestive heart failure exacerbations. *Archives of Internal Medicine*, **161**, 2337–2342.

20. van der Wal, M.H.L., Jaarsma, T. and van Veldhuisen, D.J. (2004) Non-compliance in patients with heart failure: how can we manage it? *European Journal of Heart Failure*, **7**, 5–17.

21. Huerta, C., Varas-lorenzo, C., Castellsague, J. and Rodriguez, L.A.G. (2006) Nonsteroidal anti-inflammatory drugs and risk of first hospital admission for heart failure in the general population. *Heart*, **92**, 1610–1615.

22. Ezekowitz, J.A., McAlister, F.A. and Armstrong, P.W. (2003) Anaemia is common in heart failure and is associated with poor outcomes: insights from a cohort of 12065 patients with new-onset heart failure. *Circulation*, **107**, 223–225.

23. Felker, G.M., Gattis, W.A., Leimberger, J.D., Adams, K.F. *et al.* (2003) Usefulness of anaemia as a predictor of death and rehospitalisation in patients with decompensated heart failure. *American Journal of Cardiology*, **92**, 625–628.

24. Bueno, H., Martinez-Selles, M., Perez-David, E. and Lopez-Palop, R. (2005) Effect of thrombolytic therapy on the risk of cardiac rupture and mortality in older patients with first acute myocardial infarction. *European Heart Journal*, **26**, 1705–1711.

25. de Boer, M.J., Ottervanger, J.P., van't Hof, A.W., Hoorntje, J.C. *et al.* (2002) Zwolle Myocardial Infarction Study Group. Reperfusion therapy in elderly patients with acute myocardial infarction: a randomized comparison of primary angioplasty and thrombolytic therapy. *Journal of the American College of Cardiology*, **39**, 1723–1728.

26. Dzavik, V., Sleeper, L.A., Cocke, T.P., Moscucci, M. *et al.* (2003) SHOCK Investigators. Early revascularization is associated with improved survival in elderly patients with acute myocardial infarction complicated by cardiogenic shock: a report from the SHOCK Trial Registry. *European Heart Journal*, **24**, 828–837.

27. Dzavik, V. and Hochman, J.S. (2002) Cardiogenic shock in the elderly: medical treatment or PCI? *American College of Cardiology Current Journal Review*, **11** (5), 62–66.

28. Cleland, J.G.F., Coletta, A.P., Abdellah, A.T. *et al.* (2008) Clinical trials update from the American Heart Association 2007: CORONA, RethinQ, MASCOT, AF-CHF, HART, MASTER, POISE and stem cell therapy. *European Journal of Heart Failure*, **10**, 102–108.

29. SHEP Cooperative Research Group (1991) Prevention of stroke by antihypertensive drug treatment in older persons with isolated systolic hypertension. Final results of the Systolic Hypertension in the Elderly Program (SHEP). *Journal of the American Medical Association*, **265**, 3255–3263.

30. Tribouilloy, C., Rusinaru, D., Mahjoub, H., Souliere, V. *et al.* (2008) Prognosis of heart failure with preserved ejection fraction: a 5 year prospective population-based study. *European Heart Journal*, **29**, 339–347.

31. Aronow, W.S., Ahn, C. and Kronzon, I. (1990) Prognosis of congestive heart failure in elderly patients with normal versus abnormal left ventricular systolic function associated with coronary artery disease. *American Journal of Cardiology*, **66**, 1257–1259.

32. Shahar, E., Lee, S., Kim, J. *et al.* (2004) Hospitalised heart failure: rates and long-term mortality. *Journal of Cardiac Failure*, **10**, 374–379.

33. Haldeman, G.A., Croft, J.B., Giles, W.H. *et al.* (1995) Hospitalisation of patients with heart failure: National Hospital Discharge Survey, 1985 to 1995. *American Heart Journal*, **137**, 352–360.

34. Setoguchi, S., Stevenson, L.W. and Schneeweis, S. (2007) Repeat hospitalisations predict mortality in the community population with heart failure. *American Heart Journal*, **154**, 260–266.

35. Gohler, A., Januzzi, J.L., Worrell, S.S., Osterziel, K.J. *et al.* (2006) A systematic meta-analysis of the efficacy and heterogeneity of disease management programs in congestive heart failure. *Journal of Cardiac Failure*, **12**, 554–567.

36. Fonarow, G.C., Stevenson, L.W., Walden, J.A., Livingston, N.A. *et al.* (1997) Impact of a comprehensive heart failure management program on hospital readmission and functional status of patients status of patients with advanced heart failure. *Journal of the American College of Cardiology*, **30**, 725–732.

37. Linne, A.B., Liedholm, H. and Israelsson, B. (1999) Effects of systematic education on heart failure patients' knowledge after 6 months. A randomised, controlled trial. *European Journal of Heart Failure*, **1**, 219–227.

38. Shah, M.R., Flavell, C.M., Weintraub, J.R., Young, M.A. *et al.* (2005) Intensity and focus of heart failure disease management after hospital discharge. *American Heart Journal*, **149**, 715–721.

39. Krumholz, H.M., Butler, J., Miller, J., Vaccarino, V. *et al.* (1997) Prognostic importance of emotional support for elderly patients hospitalised with heart failure. *Circulation*, **97**, 958–964.

40. Wang, L. (2007) Fundamentals of intrathoracic impedance monitoring in heart failure. *American Journal of Cardiology*, **99** (Suppl), 3G–10G.

13

Models of care and disease management programmes

Martin Wilson[1] and Stephen J. Leslie[2]

[1]Care of the Elderly, Raigmore Hospital, Inverness
[2]Cardiac Unit, Raigmore Hospital, Inverness

Key messages

- A disease management programme is a multidisciplinary approach to the care of patients throughout the course of their disease.

- Comorbidities make the provision of care more complex for older patients than for those who are younger.

- What constitutes an appropriate model of care is dependent on the expertise and facilities available locally, and will vary between urban and rural populations.

- Good communication between health care professionals and with patients is central to good disease management.

13.1 Introduction

The care of heart failure patients mostly takes place in the community and primary care. Hospital visits may be necessary as an outpatient for specialist review and investigation, while admission to hospital may be required for invasive therapies, such as cardiac resynchronization therapy (CRT), implantable cardioverter defibrillator (ICD) or treatment of clinical deteriorations. The term 'disease management

A Practical Guide to Heart Failure in Older People, Edited by C Ward and M D Witham
© 2009 John Wiley & Sons, Ltd

Table 13.1 Typical features of a patient with heart failure.

Average age at diagnosis 75 years
Poor mobility and social support
Polypharmacy
Comorbidities
Persistent symptoms
Limited knowledge of own condition
Frequent admissions to hospital

programme' refers to a comprehensive multidisciplinary approach to the care of patients. This involves patient care throughout the course of their disease process and across the breadth of the health care services, including medical, nursing and social care. There will be variation between geographical areas as to how this care is provided; for example, the model of care for congestive heart failure (CHF) may vary greatly between rural and urban populations. In addition to this, the local models or clinical pathways will depend on the availability and organization of local services, funding, geography and local facilities such as equipment, hospitals and suitably skilled staff.

The provision of care for older adults with heart failure raises further complex issues. Older adults are at higher risk of deterioration and are more likely to have comorbidities which can make the treatment of CHF more complex (Table 13.1). This group therefore may have more to gain from specialist review. Paradoxically, as older patients are more likely to be frail, travelling long distances to specialist clinics may be less practical and therefore they may be less likely to see a specialist. This appears to happen in practice, as heart failure patients who are reviewed by cardiologists compared with general physicians tend to be younger and to have fewer comorbidities [1].

Which model of care will work in a specific geographical area will depend heavily on local circumstances. It is likely that in order to improve the overall care of patients with CHF, a comprehensive tailored model of care will be required for each area reflecting local circumstances. The potential components of these models of care for heart failure patients are discussed in this chapter. None of these components, however, works effectively in isolation. Good communication is vital to providing good quality care. There is increasing evidence that a multidisciplinary team approach – most commonly led by a specialist nurse – is the best model, although which patients have most to gain from this model is less certain [2]. Furthermore, not all patients will be under the care of a heart failure nurse and therefore any disease management programme should attempt to provide equitable care by ensuring that clear care pathways are available to all health care professionals who may treat patients with heart failure, ensuring multiple access points to the various components of any model of care.

Communication

Good communication at each interface in a disease management programme is important, as poor communication is likely to lead to a reduced quality of service and often potentially dangerous drug errors. The classic example of breakdown in communication is the often poor interface between primary and secondary care, with hand-written and often inaccurate immediate discharge summaries and delayed formal discharge letters. The computerization of discharge summaries and the use of e-mail and electronic referral pathways may help in this regard. However, the increasing use of CHF specialist nurses will also facilitate safe early discharge from hospital and improve communication between primary and secondary care (see Chapter 10).

Patients report several communication issues in relation to their heart failure management, including a lack of education, psychosocial care and communication between primary and secondary care [3]. Several barriers have been identified that contribute to poor communication between doctors and patients with heart failure. These include misconceptions on the part of both patients and staff, difficulty attending hospital, and uncertainty with prognosis [4]. Good communication may be even more difficult in older patients due to specific comorbidities such as poor eyesight, deafness or cognitive impairment [5]. Older adults are also in general looked after by health professionals who are often decades younger than they are; hence, values and expectations can reasonably be expected to be considerably different. The early identification of these issues will help to avoid miscommunication.

How do we assess models of care and disease management programmes?

The most effective model of care would appear to be one which involves a co-ordinated multidisciplinary team approach, ideally led by a specialist nurse [2]. The role of the specialist nurse is described in more detail in Chapter 10. This particular model has been shown in randomized controlled trials to be effective at reducing admissions to hospital and in improving the use of evidence-based therapies, with a high level of patient satisfaction [2]. However, outcome measures such as the 'use of evidence-based therapies', 'reduced hospitalizations' and indeed 'mortality', may not be appropriate outcome measures in the older patient, particularly for those who are extremely old or frail. Outcomes based on the quality of life (including at the end of life) may be more useful measures, but are difficult to quantify and fewer data are available on specific models of CHF care in the frail older patient.

In this chapter we will discuss the various components of disease management programmes and supporting evidence, where it exists. These components may

Table 13.2   Potential elements of a CHF disease management programme.

Hospital-based care
Day hospitals
Day-care centres
Care in the community
CHF community nurse
Patient forums/carer forums/newsletters
Telemedicine
Pharmacy
Respite care
Hospice/palliative care
Family carers
Voluntary sector

include hospital-based care, day hospitals, day-care centres, heart failure nurses, telemedicine, patient and carer issues, pharmacy, palliative care, family carers and the voluntary sector (Table 13.2).

13.2   Disease management programmes

Making a diagnosis

In general, there is underdiagnosis of heart failure in the population, although overdiagnosis based on 'a clinical diagnosis only' may be a particular problem in older patients who may be unable to access diagnostic tests. An accurate identification of patients with heart failure is vital to the provision of good quality care, as many patients with left ventricular systolic dysfunction (LVSD) will be asymptomatic, while others with signs and symptoms of heart failure will have a preserved left ventricular (LV) function. The most widely used investigation for the identification of LVSD is echocardiography (Chapter 5). Access to echocardiography may be difficult for many patients, and especially those who are older. Not only is there an insufficient provision of echocardiography services in secondary care (usually due to a lack of trained sonographers), but in the older patients – and particularly those who are frail and who live a significant distance away – travel to hospital may also be impractical. Given the development of portable echocardiography machines, however, domiciliary or community echocardiography is possible [6].

Increasing the diagnostic 'suspicion' of LVSD by the use of screening tests such as electrocardiogram (ECG) and plasma levels of B-type natriuretic peptide (BNP) is encouraged in most recent guidelines [7–9]. However, the ECG interpretative skills of nonspecialists is variable [10], and although transmission to specialists is possible [11] and may improve diagnostic accuracy, logistically this is not always feasible in clinical practice. Nevertheless, the ECG is an important tool when screening for cardiac disease. Demonstrating evidence of previous myocardial infarction, atrial fibrillation and other rhythm disturbances may have important implications for the treatment of patients. This is particularly important in older patients when these conditions may be initially clinical silent but nevertheless important to detect. Given the high incidence of cardiac disease in older patients and the noninvasive nature and relative low cost of an ECG, an argument could be made for the routine ECG screening of older patients [12]. However, other studies have suggested that routine screening in an over-65-year-old population for atrial fibrillation is not cost-effective, although the opportunistic screening of such patients may be [13].

Elevated plasma concentrations of BNP and its precursor pro-N terminal BNP (pro-NT-BNP) are found in conditions which cause cardiac stress. The utility of BNP and pro-NT-BNP as a screening test for heart failure has been demonstrated in a number of clinical settings, including outpatients [14], as a guide to therapy titration in heart failure programmes [15]. Furthermore, BNP is a predictor of patients at risk of future cardiac events [16]. BNP has a high negative predictive value; that is, heart failure is unlikely in a patient with a low plasma BNP level. However, the cost-effectiveness of this approach remains controversial, and despite having been available in the UK for many years plasma BNP level has not gained widespread use as a clinical test. Which tests or combination of tests (BNP, ECG or echocardiography) will prove most cost-effective is unknown, and indeed this is likely to vary between geographical areas [17]. Clear local guidelines for primary care physicians regarding the use of these tests and subsequent pathways of care are vital to ensuring consistent good-quality care. The specifics of these disease management programmes may vary greatly between regions (Figures 13.1–13.3).

- Prehospital screen tests include ECG, BNP and echocardiography, and will vary between areas (Figures 13.1 and 13.3).

- The rapidity of access to a clinic will vary. In one area a rapid clinic exists (Figure 13.1), while in another area echocardiography guides the general practitioner (GP)-led treatment in advance of a clinical review (Figure 13.3).

- The use of community-based nurses with home visits compared to hospital-based, nurse-led clinics will depend on local circumstances; little evidence exists to favour either approach.

- Formal discharge from a heart failure service will vary between areas in agreement with local primary care services. Most disease management programmes would allow for easy re-entry into a heart failure service in response to clinical deterioration.

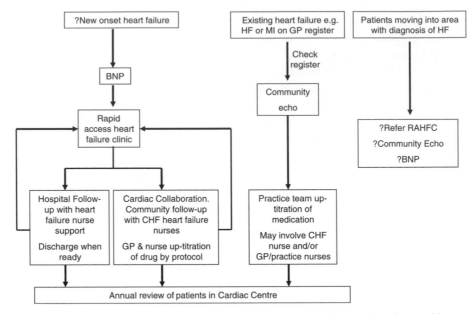

Figure 13.1   Disease management programme based on the Hastings and Rother Rapid Access Heart Failure Clinic.

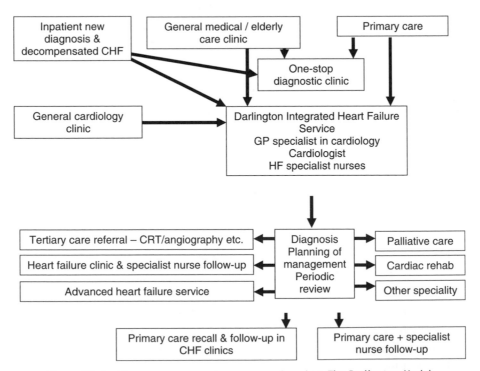

Figure 13.2   Disease management programme based on The Darlington Model.

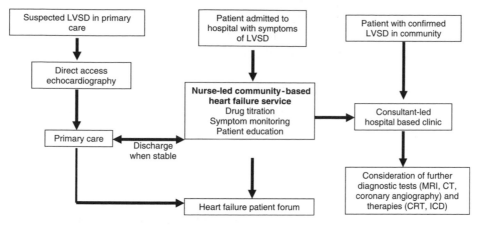

Figure 13.3 Disease management programme based on the Highland Heart Failure Service.

- Close multi-agency communication is vital to all disease management programmes.

- Referral pathways to palliative care and advanced heart failure services should be encouraged.

Once patients are referred for echocardiography, they may be treated by either primary or secondary care physicians, depending on several factors including the severity of the LVSD, symptoms and the local availability of specialist services; however, older patients are less likely to see a cardiologist [1]. One issue which is of particular difficulty is the availability of skilled staff. Even simple investigations such as an ECG require skilled interpretation if diagnostic accuracy is to be achieved. Services such as echocardiography require skilled technicians or doctors, while other investigations such as magnetic resonance may be prohibitively expensive for general widespread use in cardiac patients.

Hospital-based care

Tertiary care

Certain heart failure services are centralized in tertiary centres, including transplantation, pacemaker therapy, CRT, implantation of cardioverter defibrillator (ICD) and revascularization, although increasingly specialist services are provided in district general hospitals. Due to increased frailty, comorbidities and decreased life expectancy, older patients may be less likely to be referred to a tertiary centre. Furthermore, if patients are not seen by their local cardiologists then they are less likely to be referred for tertiary services. While therapies such as heart transplantation may be contraindicated in older patients, other therapies such as CRT and ICD improve outcome in such cases [18–21]. Clinical decisions regarding referral to a tertiary centre base on age alone should be challenged.

Secondary/district general hospital care

Hospital-based care is discussed in more detail in Chapters 11 and 12. However, appropriate discharge planning and good communication between the multidisciplinary members of a disease management programme are vital to the care of CHF patients:

- Good-quality, written and legible discharge summaries are important; an early (<1 week) follow-up by the CHF community nurse following discharge will reduce the likelihood of unnecessary readmission to hospital.

- Accurate prescribing is a key feature if admission to hospital has occurred. There are many potential sources of error, both at the time of admission and at discharge, with drug treatments being inadvertently started or stopped.

- During any hospital stay, an effort should be made to ensure that what was recorded as a patient's routine medication was accurate.

- Discharge notification should be specific about what changes to each specific medication have been made. If at all possible, a copy of the patient's primary care summary should be obtained to ensure that the medication information (including intolerances) is accurate.

- Hospital admission can be used as a chance to summarize a patient's condition and current function.

- Consideration should be given to copying the final discharge notification to the patient as a further method of ensuring they understand what has happened. This also provides a 'safety net', as a patient may be best placed to point out an error if it has occurred.

- Again, this is best supported by a heart failure nurse or other professional who can explain terms as needed.

Local or cottage hospital care

Particularly in remote and rural areas, but also in urban centres, older patients may be admitted to primary care-run Community Hospitals. This may in many ways be much less traumatic as the distances travelled can be significantly shorter and the stay itself may be more stable (missing many of the unpleasant aspects of acute hospital care such as decanting through multiple wards). There may well also be advantages in terms of continuity of care, with the same GP practice and community health partnership or primary care trust being responsible throughout. It is important, however, to ensure that older adults are not subtly disadvantaged by admission to such units. This can be done by ensuring that these units also benefit from access to all aspects of the disease management programmes, such as CHF nurses and echocardiography. Protocols for the management of acute exacerbations of heart failure can be shared between primary and secondary care to ensure equivalence between the different facilities. Occasional 'teach and treat'-style cardiology clinics in peripheral areas are one way of improving management for adults living in these areas. This could involve a traditional clinic-based assessment of patients but also include a teaching element, perhaps by discussing cases recently managed in that hospital.

Community-based care

General practice

Most treatment changes in patients with CHF are initiated or undertaken by GPs [22]. However, secondary care facilities are required for the initial diagnosis and advanced treatment. Several barriers to good CHF management exist, including a lack of confidence in general practice with drug therapy, a poor availability of diagnostic services and a lack of interaction between primary and secondary care [23] (see Chapter 8). Strategies that encourage and improve interaction between primary and secondary care (such as the 'teach and treat'-style clinics suggested above for remote areas) should be explored.

Further improvements in CHF care have been made by creating financial incentives to improve care given to patients by GPs. In the UK, the general medical services contract has succeeded in increasing the number of patients who have an echocardiogram and who are prescribed an ACE inhibitor, but clearly there is much more that could be achieved [24]

Day hospitals

Day hospitals in various forms have existed for many years, mostly in urban centres. They aim to provide a comprehensive assessment of older patients in a community setting; that is, to assess and, where needed, to rehabilitate and manage patients without recourse to hospital admission. Day hospitals can provide an opportunity for the multidisciplinary assessment of patients with heart failure and, unlike a specialist heart failure clinic, is better placed to assess comorbidities. The medical input to these units tends to be from geriatric practitioners or GPs. Although very few robust data are available to support this model in terms of reduced admissions to hospital or mortality, there does appear to be an improvement in quality of life and treatment adherence [25]. Importantly, older heart failure patients may well have this as only one item on a list of pathologies, all of which need to be dealt with and balanced in order to obtain the best outcome for that adult (see Chapter 8). Pathologies other than heart failure may well be noted particularly by CHF nurses, and a link with a local day hospital may prove a useful way to ensure that these assessment needs are met. An example is a physiotherapy/occupational therapy assessment for walking aids if the patient's mobility is reduced due to arthritis or previous stroke. It is important to note that a key feature of day hospital facilities appears to be assessment by a multidisciplinary team, including medical input. Day hospitals have been shown to effective at maintaining function, but do not necessarily have any advantage over the same comprehensive assessment strategies provided in other ways for example at home [26].

Nursing homes and care homes

When care at home becomes impractical, older patients may move to a nursing or care home. Not surprisingly, these patients will be older, more frail, have more comorbidities and have a higher mortality that the general heart failure population [27–29]. These patients are also more frequently hospitalized, which is perhaps less well-defined. It could be envisaged that, with better care in nursing homes and planning regarding end-of-life issues, admission to hospital from nursing and care homes would be reduced. Regular attendance by geriatricians to care homes appears to improve the management of older patients with heart failure [30]. Whether performed by geriatrician or GP, patients in care homes should undergo intermittent and comprehensive assessment to ensure that, as they progress through each of the later stages of their life, management decisions on the appropriateness of active treatment is reviewed and where possible discussed with the patient themselves and with those close to them.

It is likely that there is scope to improve the care of patients in nursing homes in terms of access to diagnostic tests and specialist advice. In care homes, educational procedures should include carers where possible. For example, education during the early signs of decompensation (seen as weight gain, increased oedema), supported by a management plan of what to do in this situation, would be expected to improve care. At an organizational level, ensuring that staff and out-of-hours services have access to accurate and up-to-date information on a patient's diagnosis and management will in turn help to ensure that out-of-hours care does not unnecessarily default to hospital admission [31, 32].

Heart failure nurses

The role of the heart failure nurse is described in detail in Chapter 10. In the context of disease management programmes, these nurses often provide the key role of

Table 13.3 Role of a chronic heart failure specialist nurse.

Facilitate hospital discharge
Home visit
Ensure evidence-based pharmacological treatments
Patient education
Patient and carer education and support
Weight control
Dietary measures for example salt avoidance
Reducing fluid intake
Smoking cessation
Exercise/rehabilitation
Influenza vaccination annually
Advocate for patients needs
Coordination of care
Close monitoring of U + Es
Facilitate access to hospital services
Coronary revascularization (PCI/CABG)
Cardiac resynchronization therapy (CRT)
Implantable cardioverter defibrillator (ICD)
End-of-life support
Discharge
Telephone advice helpline

coordinating other services [2], in particular providing an excellent link between primary and secondary care. Indeed, home visits by the heart failure nurse of patients recently discharged from hospital may also reduce numbers of readmissions [2]. Currently however, the majority of patients who have heart failure will not be under the care of a heart failure nurse, nor of a formal heart failure service. Disease management programmes must therefore enable multiple access points to the services that are required, and must recognize the different pathways that exist in CHF patient care, allowing equitable access to CHF services for all patients (Table 13.3).

Rehabilitation

Exercise-based rehabilitation has been shown to improve functional ability and objective measures of cardiac function [33, 34]. However, insufficient public funding of cardiac rehabilitation, at least in the UK, has resulted in a very patchy delivery of these services. There is also evidence that an invitation to exercise-based rehabilitation is more likely to be taken up by fitter, younger male patients who perhaps have less to gain than those who are older and infirm. Several barriers exist to the provision of exercise-based cardiac rehabilitation for patients with heart failure. Not least of these is the lack of provision of local classes. In older patients there are mobility issues which may make travel to classes difficult. More importantly, there may be a perception among older patients and their families that exercise- or gym-based rehabilitation is not appropriate. Yet crucially, older patients would appear to gain similar benefits than younger people from exercise [35], despite being under-represented in both clinical research studies [36] and in cardiac rehabilitation classes.

Pharmacy

As discussed in Chapter 6, the pharmacological treatment of heart failure is complex, requiring a gradual titration of drugs and flexibility depending on clinical response. there is often also a need for significant changes to the medication when there is clinical deterioration. Older patients are also more likely to have significant comorbidities which themselves will necessitate complex treatment regimes; hence, there is a high risk of polypharmacy and significant drug interactions and side effects. Safe pharmacy requires good communication between those making treatment changes (patients, doctors, nurses) and pharmacy services to avoid dangerous polypharmacy. Specific issues such as drug formulations, the timing of dosing and delivery become increasingly important in elderly patients who may find concordance with drug therapies difficult due to comorbidities (e.g. poor vision, cognitive impairment). Effective and timely communication between primary and secondary care and pharmacy is crucial to avoid treatment errors. Devices such as 'dosette boxes' are more commonly used in older patients.

Hospice/palliative care

Recently, there has been an increased focus on end-of-life issues for CHF patients, and these are discussed in Chapter 14.

Family carers

Patients of all ages with long-term conditions frequently require care. A recent survey in Scotland suggested that 11% of adults with a long-term condition have home care. A large proportion of these carers are unpaid, and most often are family members [37]. It is estimated that, in Scotland, one in eight (12–14%) of all households contain an adult who is also a carer, and that in one-third of cases this carer is the only carer for that adult. In the majority of cases (70%) where the carer lives in the house, they feel that they provide continuous care. Most often, the carer is a spouse (56%), and less frequently a son or daughter (25%). If the carer comes from outside the patient's house, he or she is most likely to be a child of the patient (61%) [38].

Carers are likely to benefit greatly from education regarding the illness and treatment of the patient, and they would reasonably be best placed to spot the subtle signs of early decompensation. They are also well placed to help patients follow self-management plans, for example increasing diuretic intake for increasing oedema or cutting back in the case of dehydration. It is the experience of both present authors that carers, as well as the patients themselves, can often become expert in the care and management of heart failure patients. In fact, in some cases they may even be better than the professionals due to their better knowledge of the particular details of the patient concerned!

Ensuring that carers are aware of what help is available should help to avoid crisis [39]. Specific examples include the development of information packs regarding what benefits are available, and what processes need to be followed if the care that a patient requires exceeds (or, as importantly, is approaching) the limit at which informal carers can cope. The logical rule here is to try and ensure that whatever simple pre-emptive measures can be taken have been taken.

Shifts in population, with the tendency for families to be spread widely in geographical terms, seems likely over time to reduce the number of people cared for by their own families. Despite many surveys having been conducted, it remains unclear at present just how many people depend on informal support. Acknowledging the benefit and hard work of informal unpaid carers can help to highlight the difficult problems of older patients isolated from their family, or living alone. It is particularly important that this group is able to access help when needed.

Patient forums/carer forums/newsletters and the voluntary sector

Many local groups provide support to heart failure patients, including both patient and carer groups. These can serve as an excellent resource for patients and health professionals alike. In particular, educational material can be very well distributed through such groups, with local and national newsletters and pamphlets offering considerable guidance and providing further sources of information. There are many local and national voluntary organizations which can offer additional support to heart failure patients and, ideally, these services should be as integrated into disease management programmes. National organizations in the UK include the British Heart Foundation and Chest Heart and Stroke Scotland. While these organizations can provide general support and information, several specific additional services exist including respite and befriending services. Although robust evidence to support the use of these services is lacking, anecdotal evidence suggests that they are greatly valued by both patients and carers.

13.3   Disease management programmes: the evidence

A recent meta-analysis of 36 randomized trials (8341 patients) provided support for disease management programmes by showing a reduction of 8% in rehospitalization and a 3% reduction in mortality ($\sim$6 months) [40]. An earlier meta-analysis of 27 randomized studies in older people (mean age $>$70 years) demonstrated an even greater impact, showing that disease management programmes in older patients could reduce readmissions for heart failure by 30%, and readmission or death by 18% ($>$6 months) [41]. Although well designed, many of these studies involved small numbers of patients, and therefore specific conclusions on efficacy of different disease management programmes, especially in the older patients, are difficult to draw.

Indeed, there is much heterogeneity between studies in terms of design and intervention, although there appears to be no significant difference in the treatment effect between interventions studied [41]. Therefore, uncertainty remains as to which specific model or disease management programme offers the best outcomes. Nevertheless, despite significant differences between programmes, most have several key features in common, including patient education, a coordinator (usually a heart failure nurse), telephone support and monitoring of symptoms and physical findings. Therefore, in the selected patients who are entered into trials, the benefits seen are most likely to be due to the common elements of these programmes (patient education, self-directed disease monitoring and close attention to changes in symptoms or physical findings). However, whether these benefits would be seen in all patients with heart failure outside the setting of a clinical trial is uncertain. Further research is clearly required to determine which patients respond best to which model.

The shared components of most successful disease management programmes include:

- A comprehensive discharge strategy
- Multiple access points to each component of the model of care
- Telephonic support
- A programme coordinator, ideally a specialist nurse.

13.4 Guidelines and critical care pathways

Critical care pathways, protocols and guidelines have become an everyday feature of clinical practice. In conditions such as heart failure, the guidelines can be complex and treatment decisions may rely heavily on clinical findings and investigations. A combination of knowledge and expert advice in addition to guidelines is therefore required for the optimal treatment of these patients. Thus, diagnosis and management of heart failure in primary care remains difficult (see Chapter 9). A number of barriers to improving heart failure services have been identified among family physicians; these include uncertainty about diagnosis, a lack of awareness of relevant research evidence, a lack of diagnostic resources such as echocardiography, and a lack of access to specialist advice [23]. The latter point may be particularly relevant in remote and rural areas, where there are considerable distances between the patients and specialist centres, making clinic review more difficult. This is compounded in some health care systems by a relative lack of specialists (e.g. the National Health Service in the UK).

Critical care pathways or guidelines represent a distillation of the best available evidence, and should improve patient management. Recently, however, guidelines have become lengthy and complex [7–9]. The impact of such documents in secondary care is suboptimal [1, 42], and in primary care it is unknown. One recognized problem is that the majority of guidelines provide broad advice on pharmacological and non-pharmacological strategies, but are unable to provide patient-specific management advice. Specific advice is often required by generalists in complex cases with multiple comorbidities, where the treatment itself may have resulted in significant problems such as renal impairment, gout or symptomatic hypotension. Previous studies have suggested that guidelines combined with expert advice from heart failure specialists represents a way of providing tailored management [43].

Clinical decision support software

Clinical decision support software (CDSS) may be able to provide such advice and support, especially when using web-based programming that allows for complex interactive page design [44]. In this particular decision support software for heart failure, users are asked to enter various clinical parameters on the left-hand side of the screen, while 'information' is generally displayed on the right-hand side of the screen (Figure 13.4). The decision support software is divided into several sections: diagnosis; drug treatment; referral; common problems; non-pharmacological advice; information for patients; and current research studies. Each of these sections has various subsections. For example, the diagnosis section asks for various clinical parameters including symptoms and signs of heart failure, past medical history and simple baseline investigations. These inputs will generate a suggestion as to the likelihood of a diagnosis of heart failure. The section on drug treatment expands to cover all commonly prescribed drug classes for heart failure; inputs are required to ensure that the drug is appropriate for use in the particular patient, and practical advice given about its initiation, up-titration (if appropriate) and common problems that may be encountered. Other sections include patient information, including

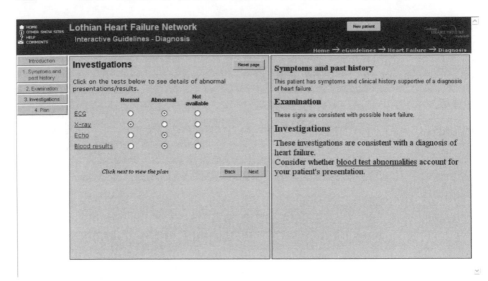

Figure 13.4   Sample page from the CDSS – 'Diagnosing heart failure'. The inputs are single mouse clicks on the left side of the page, resulting in outputs (clinical advice) on the right side of the screen.

advice about non-pharmacological issues in heart failure such as exercise and the regional heart failure newsletter.

Heart failure represents a challenging topic for decision support software development, given the large evidence base and the relatively high prevalence and complexity of social and medical management issues in both secondary and primary care. Previous computerized guidelines in heart failure have proved difficult to integrate into clinical practice and did not adequately deal with comorbidity, concurrent drug therapy or timing of interventions and follow-up [43]. However, more recently decision support software has proved useful in other conditions such as hypertension [45] and cardiovascular risk management [46]. Any computer decision support software also has the advantage that it can be easily adapted to reflect local pathways of care and referral, hopefully improving patient flow and care.

Barriers to the implementation of computerized guidelines and pathways

Poor computer skills is a barrier to implementation, especially among family physicians. This must be carefully considered and accounted for within the design, since previous studies have suggested that decision support software available for use during patient consultations may be disruptive [47]. However, it is clear that medical students and junior doctors – as the next generation of health care professionals – may bring a higher level of computer literacy to the clinical arena [44]. This is likely to help the implementation of decision support software in the future. Additionally, integration of the program into routine clinical practice may also help with features such as automatic referral letter generation. This design feature of a 'referral letter' or 'echocardiography request' incorporated into an electronic guideline is one way of ensuring a wider use of clinical decision support software.

13.5 Remote and rural issues

Increased geographical remoteness leads to reduced access to centralized specialist services. This occurs for one of two reasons: (i) services and staff are centralized, making travel to the centre a barrier; or (ii) a peripheral (local) service is offered by a visiting specialists, but because of travel time and smaller number of patients, this becomes either a less efficient or a more expensive model of care delivery. It would appear, however, that while patients are prepared to travel to a specialist service for 'one-off' therapies, they prefer a local service for recurrent appointments. There-fore, patients might expect to travel to have a pacemaker or ICD implant, but would prefer a local delivery of cardiac rehabilitation or drug titration. In a remote area, some part of the heart failure service may need to be devolved to other individuals, for example community nurses rather than heart failure nurses, or the GP rather than hospital physicians (Table 13.4). In remote areas with small populations, education of the care providers should be a major focus. Letters from secondary care following initial assessment and diagnosis should be particularly clear as to the current steps in treatment and drug titration. Also included could be standard advice on 'Frequently Asked Questions' on a pre-emptive basis; for example, What to do if a patient on heart failure drugs coincidently gets

Table 13.4 Potential differences between rural and urban heart failure services.

	Urban	Rural
Diagnostics		
BNP	Not cost-effective compared to ECG alone?	May prevent travel to hospital if limited access to ECG
Diagnostics (e.g. echocardiography)	Hospital-based	Visiting service (Road Show)
Treatment		
Clinics	Greater reliance on hospital clinics	More GP-based
HF nurses	More direct care	More advisory
Telemedicine		More likely to be cost-effective

gastroenteritis? Support to health professionals in these areas needs to make as much use as possible of the telephone, e-mail and telemedicine as possible, in order to ensure that treatment gradients that are recognized as being as small as possible [48]. The aim should be to make access to advice as simple as possible, encouraging questions that may seem to be too simple to warrant a long journey to a hospital clinic. Typical questions would relate to drug titration, side effects, or when to add in further medication.

13.6   Telecardiology in heart failure

Telecardiology may include a variety of devices aimed at improving patient care. These can range from simple techniques for collecting clinical data without the need for face-to-face consultation, to sophisticated telemonitoring systems and even complex therapy changes (e.g. remote pacemaker reprogramming) (Table 13.5).

Home telemonitoring has recently been the focus of considerable investment, and has been seen as an opportunity to reduce hospital admissions by increasing stability in the home environment. These technologies potentially have great utility in patients with heart failure, who often have a gradual deterioration in their clinical state before requiring admission to hospital. There is therefore potential for the early identification of patients who may be at risk of significant clinical deterioration requiring hospitalization. Furthermore, the use of such systems might increase the compliance of patients with home monitoring of weight and symptoms, and may enable patients to take a more active role in their own disease management, including concordance with medications. However, some home monitoring technologies require considerable commitment from patients and also support for their use in terms of the interface with the patient, IT support for the transmission of information to the monitoring centre, and the development of agreed local protocols.

Considerable thought and planning is required to have robust protocols in the event of a change in the patient's clinical state, and this will require locality specific protocols with the agreement of local practitioners – and therefore 'one size' will not 'fit all'.

Table 13.5 Potential benefits of telemedicine.

Reduced visits to hospital
Improved communication between patients/GP/secondary care
Improved data transfer and monitoring
Reduced hospitalizations?

Even with an optimal design of individual telemonitoring systems, some patients will not be able nor prepared to utilize this technology. This may in particular be pertinent to older patients where comorbidities such as poor vision, deafness, dementia and, not least, relatively lesser IT skills may make telemonitoring impractical.

A recent review [49] identified nine randomized controlled trials investigating telemonitoring in heart failure, with outcomes that included hospitalization or mortality. Although direct comparisons between studies are difficult due to widely varying entry criteria, study design and interventions, they can broadly be divided into those studies which use mainly telephone monitoring, patient-activated devices (telemonitoring) or implantable automated devices (e.g. pacemakers).

Telephone-based monitoring

Most studies using telephone monitoring used trained nurses in live one-to-one telephone calls with patients. However, subsequent interventions vary between studies. The majority of these studies demonstrated a reduction in hospitalization [50–53], although one study showed no benefit [54]. Despite this single negative result, the majority of telephone intervention studies demonstrated benefit. Only one study performed a formal prospective cost analysis, and found telephone monitoring to be cost-effective [52]. However, the cost-efficacy of such an intervention will rely heavily on local expenditure on health care and the level of standard treatment. Indeed, a high level of quality standard therapy (USA) may explain the negative outcome of the one study noted above [54].

Telemonitoring

There are relatively few studies on telemonitoring devices. One study evaluated twice-weekly electronic home monitoring of symptoms and weight [55], with the devices being linked to a hub monitored by trained nurses. Although there was a reduction in mortality of 56%, there was no reduction in rates of hospitalization. In a further study, daily home monitoring of weight, blood pressure, heart rate and oxygen saturations (with data sent to the cardiologist) appeared to show a 40% reduction in hospitalizations compared to nurse home visits. This was a small study based in the USA which, although reported as being cost-effective, may not be applicable or cost-effective in most other health care systems. A further study conducted by Cleland *et al.* compared telemonitoring with nurse telephone support [56]. Physiological measurements were made twice weekly and reviewed by trained nurses, who could adjust the patient's medication according to protocol. The telephone calls were made monthly. Both of these interventions resulted in a trend to reduction in hospitalization and mortality; however, there was no difference between telephone calls or telemonitoring. A small study investigated the use of video conferencing or telephone support versus usual care. Again, small benefits were seen in the intervention groups, but no difference was apparent between the two approaches.

Implantable monitoring devices

Recent developments in advanced pacing and the publication of mortality data supporting the use of ICDs and CRT in patients with heart failure has led to the development of sophisticated telemonitoring through these implantable devices. A range of physiological measurements can be constantly monitored in real time and transmitted electronically. While these devices are expensive and invasive initially, they may prove less intrusive in the patients' lives. Good data management and clear clinical pathways to deal with deranged patient parameters, especially outside office hours, are required if these devices are to be clinically useful. Further studies are required to define which patient may benefit from the continuous monitoring feature of these technologies.

Telecardiology conclusions

It is difficult to draw firm conclusions regarding telemonitoring based on the limited data available. What does appear to be true is that any intervention – for example, telephone support, home visits, telemonitoring or video conferencing – appears to offer benefit in terms of reduced hospitalization and perhaps mortality. Which of these is most effective and cost-efficient remains uncertain, and whether there are specific patients groups that will gain most from each approach requires further research. It is likely that most benefit will be gained from those who are at greatest risk of hospitalization, although a very sick patient may be hospitalized regardless of intervention. Current study designs and a lack of funding, along with publication pressures to gain a positive result, might result in neglect and under-investigation of lower-risk patients with mild heart failure who nevertheless have a high lifetime risk of developing significant heart failure requiring hospitalization.

Meanwhile, there are many commercially available devices for telemonitoring of heart failure patients, although disappointingly there are few data to support their use. Health care providers and purchasers currently would have difficulty in making informed decisions based on currently available data. However, despite the lack of robust data, telemedicine is an exciting development which may find most use in dispersed populations where the long distances between specialist and patient makes regular home visits costly. In addition, these technologies will have to be used in a supported manner, which is especially important in the older patients who may be less skilled with electronic equipment.

13.7 Conclusions

A recent meeting of key stakeholders arranged by the Clinical Effectiveness and Evaluation Unit of the Royal College of Physicians concluded that in the UK [57]:

- Heart failure care varies substantially across the country.

- There are deficiencies in both the organization of care and the process of care. The best services are those which cross primary and secondary care with effective communication between the health professionals, and which involve the patient in their own management.

- Accurate diagnosis is important for correct management. Many new referrals to a heart failure service do not have heart failure.

- Good data – particularly on the outcome of care – are the exception, not the rule. Collecting data helps to both plan and deliver services.

- Good heart failure care can be delivered by the NHS, although staffing and structures will vary according to local factors.

In order to improve care for patients with heart failure there will need to be a much greater 'organization' of services. This does not necessarily mean greater central control, and indeed locally tailored disease management programmes are likely to be more successful and easier to implement that a 'one size fits all' approach. What is clear, however, is that there needs to be an increased focus on the care of patients with heart failure, and that central fiscal measures such as the National Service Framework in England and Wales, the general medical services contract in General Practice and Quality Improvement Scotland, do have the potential to improve patient care. However, current heart failure programmes appear to rely heavily on sporadic funding and local 'clinical champions', and this leads to an inequitable provision of care.

References

1. McKee, S.P., Leslie, S.J., LeMaitre, J.P. *et al.* (2003) Management of chronic heart failure due to systolic left ventricular dysfunction by cardiologist and non-cardiologist physicians. *European Journal of Heart Failure*, **5**, 549–555.
2. Blue, L., Lang, E., McMurray, J.J. *et al.* (2001) Randomised controlled trial of specialist nurse intervention in heart failure. *British Medical Journal*, **323**, 715–718.
3. Boyd, K.J., Murray, S.A., Kendall, M. *et al.* (2004) Living with advanced heart failure: a prospective, community based study of patients and their carers. *European Journal of Heart Failure*, **6**, 585–591.

4. Rogers, A.E., Addington-Hall, J.M., Abery, A.J. *et al.* (2000) Knowledge and communication difficulties for patients with chronic heart failure: qualitative study. *British Medical Journal*, **321**, 605–607.

5. Almeida, O.P. and Flicker, L. (2001) The mind of a failing heart: as systematic review of the association between congestive heart failure and cognitive functioning. *Internal Medicine Journal*, **31**, 290–295.

6. Galasko, G.I.W., Lahiri, A. and Senior, R. (2003) Portable echocardiography: an innovative toll in screening for cardiac abnormalities in the community. *European Journal of Echocardiography*, **4**, 119–127.

7. Remme, W.J. and Swedberg, K. (2002) Comprehensive guidelines for the diagnosis and treatment of chronic heart failure. Task force for the diagnosis and treatment of chronic heart failure of the European Society of Cardiology. *European Journal of Heart Failure*, **4**, 11–22.

8. National Institute of Clinical Excellence (NICE) (2003) *Management of chronic heart failure in adults in primary and secondary care*. Royal College of Physicians, London. Available at http://www.nice.org.uk/nicemedia/pdf/Full_HF_Guideline.pdf.

9. Scottish Intercollegiate Guidelines Network (2007) *Management of Chronic Heart Failure*. Royal College of Physicians, Edinburgh. Available at http://www.sign.ac.uk/guidelines/fulltext/93-97/index.html.

10. Goudie, B.M., Jarvis, R.I., Donnan, P.T. *et al.* (2007) Screening for left ventricular systolic dysfunction using GP-reported ECGs. *British Journal of General Practice*, **57**, 191–195.

11. Barclay, J.L., MacFarlane, P., Potts, S. and Leslie, S.J. (2008) Evaluation of a new device for the transmission of electrocardiograms by e-mail. *Journal of Telemedicine and Telecare*, **14**, 219–220.

12. De Ruijter, W., Westendorp, R.G., Macfarlane, P.W. *et al.* (2007) The routine electrocardiogram for cardiovascular risk stratification in old age: the Leiden 85-plus study. *Journal of the American Geriatrics Society*, **55**, 872–877.

13. Hobbs, F.D., Fitzmaurice, D.A., Mant, J. *et al.* (2005) A randomised controlled trial and cost-effectiveness study of systematic screening (targeted and total population screening) versus routine practice for the detection of atrial fibrillation in people aged 65 and over. The SAFE study. *Health Technology Assessment*, **9**, 1–74.

14. Weber, M. and Hamm, C. (2006) Role of B-type natriuretic peptide (BNP) and NT-proBNP in clinical routine. *Heart (British Cardiac Society)*, **92**, 843–849.

15. Troughton, R.W., Frampton, C.M., Yandle, T.G. *et al.* (2000) Treatment of heart failure guided by plasma aminoterminal brain natriuretic peptide (N-BNP) concentrations. *Lancet*, **355**, 1126–1130.

16. Berger, R., Huelsman, M., Strecker, K. *et al.* (2002) B-type natriuretic peptide predicts sudden death in patients with chronic heart failure. *Circulation*, **105**, 2392–2397.

17. Senior, R., Galasko, G., McMurray, J.V. and Mayet, J. (2003) Screening for left ventricular dysfunction in the community: role of hand held echocardiography and brain natriuretic peptides. *Heart (British Cardiac Society)*, **89** (Suppl III), iii24–iii28.

18. Ermis, C., Zhu, A.X., Vanheel, L. *et al.* (2007) Comparison of ventricular arrhythmia burden, therapeutic interventions, and survival, in patients <75 and patients > or = 75 years of age treated with implantable cardioverter defibrillators. *Europace*, **9**, 270–274.

19. Kron, J. and Conti, J.B. (2007) Cardiac resynchronization therapy for treatment of heart failure in the elderly. *Heart Failure Clinic*, **3**, 511–518.

20. Healey, J.S., Hallstrom, A.P., Kuck, K.H. *et al.* (2007) Role of the implantable defibrillator among elderly patients with a history of life-threatening ventricular arrhythmias. *European Heart Journal*, **28**, 1746–1749.

21. Delnoy, P.P., Ottervanger, J.P., Luttikhuis, H.O. *et al.* (2008) Clinical response of cardiac resynchronization therapy in the elderly. *American Heart Journal*, **155**, 746–751.

22. Rutten, F.H., Grobbee, D.E. and Hoes, A. (2003) Differences between general practitioners and cardiologists in diagnosis and management of heart failure: a survey in everyday practice. *European Journal of Heart Failure*, **5**, 337–344.

23. Fuat, A., Hungin, A.P.S. and Murphy, J.J. (2003) Barriers to accurate diagnosis and effective management of heart failure in primary care: qualitative study. *British Medical Journal*, **326**, 196.

24. Leslie, S.J., McKee, S.P., Imray, E.A. and Denvir, M.A. (2005) Management of chronic heart failure: perceived needs of general practitioners in light of the new general medical services contract. *Postgraduate Medical Journal*, **81**, 321–326.

25. Eagle, D.J., Guyatt, G.H., Patterson, C. *et al.* (1991) Effectiveness of a geriatric day hospital. *Canadian Medical Association Journal*, **318**, 699–704.

26. Forster, A., Young, J. and Langhorne, P. (2000) Medical day hospital care for the elderly versus alternative forms of care. *Cochrane Database of Systematic Reviews*, **2**, CD001730.

27. Wang, R., Mouliswar, M., Denman, S. and Kleban, M. (1998) Mortality of the institutionalized old-old hospitalized with congestive heart failure. *Archives of Internal Medicine*, **158**, 2464–2468.

28. Gambassi, G., Forman, D.E., Lapane, K.L. *et al.* (2000) Management of heart failure among very old persons living in long-term care: has the voice of trials spread? The SAGE Study Group. *American Heart Journal*, **139**, 85–93.

29. Valle, R., Aspromonte, N., Barro, S. *et al.* (2005) The NT-proBNP assay identifies very elderly nursing home residents suffering from pre-clinical heart failure. *European Journal of Heart Failure*, **7**, 542–551.

30. Misiaszek, B., Heckman, G.A., Merali, F. *et al.* (2005) Digoxin prescribing for heart failure in elderly residents of long-term care facilities. *Canadian Journal of Cardiology*, **21**, 281–286.

31. Litaker, J.R. and Chou, J.Y. (2003) Patterns of pharmacologic treatment of congestive heart failure in elderly nursing home residents and related issues: a review of the literature. *Clinical Therapeutics*, **25**, 1918–1935.

32. Rondinini, L., Coceani, M., Borelli, G. *et al.* (2008) Survival and hospitalization in a nurse-led domiciliary intervention for elderly heart failure patients. *Journal of Cardiovascular Medicine (Hagerstown, Md.)*, **9**, 470–475.

33. Afzal, A., Brawner, C.A. and Keteyian, S.J. (1998) Exercise training in heart failure. *Progress in Cardiovascular Diseases*, **41**, 175–190.
34. Belardinelli, R., Georgiou, D., Cianci, G. *et al.* (1999) Randomized controlled trial of long term moderate exercise training in chronic heart failure: effects on functional capacity, quality of life, and clinical outcome. *Circulation*, **99**, 1173–1182.
35. Ferrara, N., Corbi, G., Bosimini, E. *et al.* (2006) Cardiac rehabilitation in the elderly: patient selection and outcomes. *American Journal of Geriatric Cardiology*, **15**, 22–27.
36. Pasquali, S.K., Alexander, K.P. and Peterson, E.D. (2001) Cardiac rehabilitation in the elderly. *American Heart Journal*, **142**, 748–755.
37. Harkins, J. and Dudleston, A. (2006) *Scottish Household Survey Topic Report: Characteristics and Experiences of Unpaid Carers in Scotland*, Scottish Executive Publications.
38. Loretto, W. and Taylor, M. (2007) *Characteristics of adults in Scotland with long–term conditions: an analysis of Scottish household and Scottish Health surveys*, Scottish Government Social Research 2007, Scottish Executive Publications.
39. Ward, C. (2007) Improving access to financial support for heart failure patients: understanding the claims process and the doctor's role. *British Journal of Cardiology*, **14**, 275–279.
40. Göhler, A., Januzzi, J.L., Worrell, S.S., Osterziel, K.J., Gazelle, G.S., Dietz, R. and Siebert, U. (2006) A systematic meta-analysis of the efficacy and heterogeneity of disease management programs in congestive heart failure. *Journal of Cardiac Failure*, **12** (7), 554–567.
41. Gonseth, J., Guallar-Castillón, P., Banegas, J.R. and Rodríguez-Artalejo, F. (2004) The effectiveness of disease management programmes in reducing hospital re-admission in older patients with heart failure: a systematic review and meta-analysis of published reports. *European Heart Journal*, **25** (18), 1570–1595.
42. Bellotti, P., Badano, L.P., Acquarone, N. *et al.* (2001) Specialty-related differences in the epidemiology, clinical profile, management and outcome of patients hospitalized for heart failure; the OSCUR study. *European Heart Journal*, **22**, 596–604.
43. Tierney, W.M., Overhage, J.M., Takesue, B.Y. *et al.* (1995) Computerizing guidelines to improve care and patient outcomes: the example of heart failure. *Journal of the American Medical Informatics Association*, **2**, 316–322.
44. Leslie, S.J., Hartswood, M., Meurig, C. *et al.* (2006) Clinical decision support software for management of chronic heart failure: Development and evaluation. *Computers in Biology and Medicine*, **36**, 495–506.
45. Persson, M., Mjörndal, T., Carlberg, B. *et al.* (2000) Evaluation of a computer-based decision support system for treatment of hypertension with drugs: retrospective, noninterventional testing of cost and guideline adherence. *Journal of Internal Medicine*, **247**, 87–93.
46. Hingorani, A.D. and Vallance, P. (1999) A simple computer program for guiding management of cardiovascular risk factors and prescribing. *British Medical Journal*, **318**, 101–105.
47. Brownbridge, G., Evans, A., Fitter, M. and Platts, M. (1986) An interactive computerized protocol for the management of hypertension: effects on the general practitioner's behaviour. *Journal of the Royal College of General Practitioners*, **36**, 198–202.

48. Clark, R.A., Eckert, K.A., Stewart, S. *et al.* (2007) Rural and urban differentials in primary care management of chronic heart failure: new data from the CASE study. *The Medical Journal of Australia*, **186**, 441–445.

49. Chaudhry, S.I., Phillips, C.O., Stewart, S.S. *et al.* (2007) Telemonitoring for patients with chronic heart failure: a systematic review. *Journal of Cardiac Failure*, **13**, 56–62.

50. DIAL (2005) Randomised trial of telephone intervention in chronic heart failure: DIAL trial. *British Medical Journal*, **331**, 425.

51. Dunagan, W.C., Littenberg, B., Ewald, G.A. *et al.* (2005) Randomized trial of a nurse-administered, telephone-based disease management program for patients with heart failure. *Journal of Cardiac Failure*, **11**, 358–365.

52. Riegel, B., Carlson, B., Kopp, Z. *et al.* (2002) Effect of a standardized nurse case-management telephone intervention on resource use in patients with chronic heart failure. *Archives of Internal Medicine*, **162**, 705–712.

53. Riegel, B., Carlson, B., Glaser, D. and Romero, T. (2006) Randomized controlled trial of telephone case management in Hispanics of Mexican origin with heart failure. *Journal of Cardiac Failure*, **12**, 211–219.

54. DeBusk, R.F., Miller, N.H., Parker, K.M. *et al.* (2004) Care management for low-risk patients with heart failure: a randomised, controlled trial. *Annals of Internal Medicine*, **141**, 606–613.

55. Goldberg, L.R., Piette, J.D., Walsh, M.N. *et al.* (2003) Randomized trial of daily electronic home monitoring system in patients with advanced heart failure: the Weight Monitoring in Heart Failure (WHARF) trial. *American Heart Journal*, **146**, 705–712.

56. Cleland, J.G., Louis, A.A., Rigby, A.S. *et al.* (2005) Noninvasive home telemonitoring for patients with heart failure at high risk of recurrent admission and death: the Trans-European Network-Home-Care Management System (TEN-HMS) study. *Journal of the American College of Cardiology*, **45**, 1654–1664.

57. Pearson, M. Cowie, M. (eds) and the Staff of the Clinical Effectiveness and Evaluation Unit of the Royal College of Physicians (2005) *Managing Chronic Heart Failure: Learning from Best Practice (Implementing NICE/N0CC-CC Guidelines on Chronic Conditions)*, 1st edn, Royal College of Physicians, London.

14

Palliative and supportive care for patients with advanced and terminal heart failure

Christopher Ward[1], Francis G. Dunn[2], Shona M.M. Jenkins[2] and Martin Leiper[3]

[1]Ninewells Hospital and Medical School, Dundee
[2]Cardiac Department, Stobhill Hospital, Glasgow
[3]Consultant in Palliative Medicine, NHS Tayside

Key messages

- Palliative care strategies can control the physical symptoms and mental distress of heart failure patients which do not respond to conventional cardiological treatment.

- These strategies are particularly relevant to patients with advanced and terminal heart failure.

- Most of the palliative care needs of heart failure patients can be managed using basic palliative care skills; specialist advice is needed only occasionally.

- All health care professionals caring for heart failure patients should acquire basic palliative care skills.

A Practical Guide to Heart Failure in Older People, Edited by C Ward and M D Witham
© 2009 John Wiley & Sons, Ltd

14.1   What is palliative care?

Palliation means to 'cloak' or 'cover'. It is an alternative method of care and treatment that emphasizes whole-person care when disease-modifying treatment is no longer effective. It is a reasonable alternative to the purely biomedical model – and a far more acceptable model than, 'Sorry, nothing more can be done'.

The primary objective is to improve the quality of patients' lives, while acknowledging that the disease is incurable. This is achieved by focussing on those aspects of care which are often inadequately treated or are ignored by more conventional treatment strategies:

- The control of all physical symptoms, using mostly generic treatment protocols.

- Communicating openly with patients and carers. This includes addressing the psychological, social and 'spiritual' (not necessarily 'religious') problems which are common in patients with life-threatening illnesses.

- Helping patients, family members and other carers to cope with the impact of the patient's illness and its consequences [1].

There is still widespread misunderstanding of what palliative care can provide, and to which patients it is relevant. This can perhaps best be clarified by stating what it is not:

- It is not a cancer-specific treatment strategy, and palliative care teams do not exclusively treat cancer patients. The provision of equitable palliative care to patients without cancer is currently a priority within palliative medicine services.

- Palliative care strategies are generic and adaptable to all clinical situations.

- The aim is neither to shorten nor to increase life expectancy.

- Palliative care includes, but is not synonymous with, terminal care. In fact some aspects of palliative care, notably good communication (see below), should be introduced as a matter of course from an early stage of the disease.

- Palliative care does not replace conventional treatment, it complements it.

- Palliative care does not mean hospice care.

- Most people with heart failure can be effectively treated with generalist palliative care techniques. They do not need a specialist inpatient environment, or indeed a specialist opinion from a hospice. However, complex problems and intractable symptoms may require specialist palliative care or inpatient hospice care.

14.2 Age-related problems and the provision of palliative care

Whereas older patients may sometimes be legitimately denied optimum conventional treatment, palliative care strategies are applicable to patients of all ages. There are, however, a number of reasons why its provision may be more complicated, time-consuming and 'labour-intensive' in older patients:

- The high prevalence of comorbidities (Chapter 8) not only excludes them from some conventional treatments but also increases the need for supportive care.

- Cognitive impairment and Alzheimer's disease are common in older patients with heart failure. This increases the need for social and medical support, but makes communication more difficult and adds to the difficulties faced by carers.

- Depression is especially common in older heart failure patients and adds to their distress, but it is frequently overlooked.

- Minor problems have a greater cumulative effect on older than on younger patients, partly because of the high level of pre-existing morbidity.

- There is a tendency for inadequate assessment and under-treatment when compared to the treatment of younger patients.

- Social and financial problems are more common.

- As life expectancy increases so too does the time spent in poor health (see Chapter 2).

In this chapter we will provide an outline of the palliative care strategies which are most relevant to patients with heart failure, concentrating on those in the advanced and terminal stages of the disease as defined below. It is based largely on advice and recommendations given in UK national guidelines [2–5]. The objectives are to:

- Define the patients most in need of palliative care and summarize their conventional treatment.

- Explain why palliative support is necessary.

- Outline the appropriate strategies.

- Summarize the principles of generic symptom control.

- Provide a timetable for the introduction of palliative support.

This is not intended to be a detailed account of specialist palliative care, nor of how to manage the small number of patients with more complex problems. These details are presented in standard textbooks and in the references and other resources noted in the text.

14.3   Advanced and terminal heart failure

While some aspects of palliative care are relevant to heart failure patients throughout the disease (notably the use of communication skills to advise, inform and to discuss other issues), it is during the advanced and terminal stages of heart failure that that the provision of palliative support is most needed.

Definition and disease trajectory

Patients with advanced heart failure (HF) have documented left ventricular (LV) dysfunction and the presence of severe symptoms and poor exercise tolerance – NYHA functional Class III or IV – which have persisted for at least three months, despite attempts to optimize standard therapy [6]. As in earlier stages of the disease, many patients die suddenly and unexpectedly. Patients may remain relatively stable, although severely limited, for several months or years, but at some point the symptoms deteriorate further and become increasingly resistant to treatment. And, as time progresses, it may become appropriate or necessary to begin to withdraw conventional therapy whilst escalating palliative support; at this point the need for hospitalization because of complications or further deterioration is common. By this stage, management strategies need to include both traditional evidence-based HF treatment and various elements of palliative care.

Terminal HF may follow a gradual process of deterioration or may be precipitated by a specific event, commonly myocardial ischaemia, an arrhythmia or an infection (see Chapter 12). This terminal stage may last several days or more, during which effective palliation is of paramount importance.

Conventional management

The approach to the conventional treatment for HF is, as detailed in Chapter 6, dictated largely by guideline-based medications, including ACE inhibitors, angiotensin II receptor blockers, spironolactone and beta-blockers plus diuretics. These, with the exception of diuretics, improve both symptoms and prognosis [7–11] (Table 14.1). However, treatment may have to be modified for a variety of reasons, most of which are related to either the aetiology or comorbidities. For example, if coronary artery disease is the underlying cause (see Chapter 4), then aspirin and statins will both play a key role in survival [12, 13].

Table 14.1 Conventional treatment in advanced and terminal heart failure.

Drug	Survival improved?	Symptoms improved?	Side effects	Advanced heart failure	Terminal heart failure
ACE inhibitor	Yes	Yes	Cough	Continue except during intercurrent illness with hypovolaemia	Discontinue
		Improvement in dyspnoea, fatigue and functional capacity and reduction in hospital admissions	Hypotension	Caution in renal impairment or with other potassium sparing medication	
			Hyperkalaemia Worsening renal impairment Dizziness		
Amiodarone	No	Yes	Photosensitivity	Continue unless specific adverse effects	Discontinue
		Reduction in arrhythmia associated symptoms	Hepatic dysfunction		
			Thyroid dysfunction Nausea QT prolongation		
ARB[a]	Yes	Yes	No cough but otherwise as for ACE inhibitor	As for ACE inhibitor	Discontinue
		As for ACE inhibitor			
Aspirin	Yes	No	Gastrointestinal irritation/haemorrhage	No proven role in non-ischaemic heart failure	Discontinue

(continued)

Table 14.1 (*Continued*)

Drug	Survival improved?	Symptoms improved?	Side effects	Advanced heart failure	Terminal heart failure
Beta-blocker	Yes	Yes	Bradycardia	Continue unless thought to be contributing to fatigue	Discontinue
		As for ACE inhibitor	Hypotension Cold peripheries Nightmares Depression Fatigue Muscle weakness		
Digoxin	No	Yes	Gastrointestinal disturbance	Continue, but vigilance required to prevent toxicity. Be aware of possible drug interactions	May still provide some symptom relief in the terminal phase
		As for ACE inhibitor	Loss of appetite Agitation and depression Drowsiness and nightmares Bradycardia and heart block		
Diuretic	Probably	Yes	Dehydration	Continue with careful monitoring and adjustment of dose	May provide symptomatic benefit even in terminal heart failure

		Improvement in dyspnoea and oedema and a reduction in hospital admissions	Hypokalaemia Gout		
Hydralazine	Yes (with long-acting nitrates)	No	Gastrointestinal disturbance Headache Flushing Drug-induced lupus	Continue but only if thought to be relieving symptoms	Discontinue
Nitrates	Yes (with hydralazine)	Yes — Sublingual nitrates may lessen dyspnoea	Headache Sleep disturbance Gastrointestinal disturbance	As for Hydralazine	Discontinue
Spironolactone	Yes	Yes — Improvement in dyspnoea, fatigue and functional capacity	Hyperkalaemia Gastrointestinal disturbance Gynaecomastia	As for ACE inhibitor	Discontinue
Statin	No	No	Myalgia (rare) Hepatic dysfunction (rare) Myositis (very rare)	Stop if side effects. No proven role in nonischaemic heart failure	Discontinue

[a]Angiotensin receptor blocker.

Of equal importance is the need to adjust treatment because of renal dysfunction. This may only require a temporary adjustment, but in patients with advanced HF, as more patients develop renal dysfunction, a permanent reduction in or discontinuation of ACE inhibitors, angiotensin II receptor blockers and/or spironolactone is necessary – as a result of which the prognostic and symptomatic benefit of these drugs is lost or reduced. (With respect to diuretics, it is not entirely clear whether or not they improve the prognosis, but there is a significant body of evidence to support their efficacy in relieving breathlessness and oedema [14].)

It is also worth mentioning digoxin, the role of which has been debated. Although having no prognostic benefit, digoxin is a symptomatically beneficial agent, and as long as the patient is not experiencing any adverse effects from this, it should be continued [15].

In the past, radiofrequency ablation for dysrhythmias (in particular atrial fibrillation), cardiac resynchronization therapy (CRT) and implantable cardioverter defibrillator (ICD) were recommended in only a highly selected patient group. However, that situation is changing rapidly and these devices are now being used increasingly in advanced HF (although at present this is predominantly in younger patients) with important symptomatic benefits to the patient [16, 17]. In the case of CRT, there is also a prognostic benefit, particularly when combined with an ICD [18, 19].

14.4   Management of specific symptoms

Dyspnoea

Dyspnoea is the most common symptom in patients with advanced HF [20]. This may be debilitating both in terms of poor exercise tolerance and psychological distress. The underlying pathophysiology is complex and not fully understood, but is thought to involve increased chemoreceptor sensitivity and perfusion–ventilation mismatch in the lungs [21].

A common misperception is that dyspnoea in HF is solely a consequence of pulmonary oedema, but in fact it often persists after the patient becomes euvolaemic. It is therefore important to identify and treat any additional pathologies which may exacerbate dyspnoea. The condition may be secondary to concomitant respiratory infection, pleural effusion, pulmonary embolism or bronchial neoplasm. Atrial fibrillation and anaemia are both common in HF and may result in worsening dyspnoea. These considerations are particularly important in older patients, where multiple comorbidities are common. If the symptom of dyspnoea remains problematic when these factors have been considered and addressed, then further therapy may include supplemental oxygen, opioids or benzodiazepines.

Oxygen

In theory, supplemental inspired oxygen therapy might improve dyspnoea in advanced HF. There is, however, little objective evidence to support its use unless other factors are contributing to hypoxia, for example pulmonary oedema, a concomitant lower respiratory tract infection or chronic obstructive pulmonary disease (COPD). One small study compared cardiorespiratory responses to exercise in 12 patients with stable congestive HF and NYHA class II-III dyspnoea [22]. The results demonstrated a small, but statistically significant, improvement in oxygen saturation, exercise duration and subjective perception of dyspnoea with 50% inspired oxygen in comparison to room air. However, two subsequent small, randomized controlled trials demonstrated no physiological, functional or subjective benefit from the administration of oxygen at concentrations varying between 24 and 60% [23, 24]. While any clear objective benefits of oxygen in these patients are lacking, anecdotally, some patients with advanced HF do derive some comfort from it. Others, however, find that it causes dryness of the eyes and mouth and, as a result of the latter effect, impedes communication. Any decision to administer such therapy should therefore be tailored to each individual patient [25].

Opioids

Oral, nebulized and intravenous opioids are frequently used to ameliorate dyspnoea in patients with advanced airways disease and malignancy, and there is a fair body of evidence to support this [26]. Dyspnoea in HF is considered to be in part mediated by an augmentation of chemosensitivity [27], and so it follows that suppression of this process with opioids may improve symptoms. Intravenous morphine is commonplace in the management of acute LV failure and is often used in terminal HF during the last few days of life. However, the role of regular opioids in stable advanced HF has been assessed in only a handful of studies [28–31]. The sole study of oral morphine in advanced HF was a randomized double-blind placebo-controlled crossover study of 10 patients with stable congestive HF and NYHA class III-IV dyspnoea [29]. Oral morphine 5 mg q.i.d. or placebo was administered for four days, followed by a two-day washout period, and then crossover to the other treatment arm. Treatment with morphine was well tolerated with no significant difference in nausea, blood pressure or respiratory rate between the treatment arms. Six of the 10 patients identified a statistically significant improvement in their dyspnoea during the morphine arm, and four patients continued to take oral morphine regularly for 12 months after the study, with continued benefit. The other two patients stopped therapy due to unacceptable levels of sedation.

National and international guidelines do not specifically advocate the use of opioids in stable advanced HF, but in practice oral morphine is often prescribed.

In general, short-acting preparations are preferred due to the propensity for these patients to develop renal impairment secondary to chronic administration of diuretics and renin–angiotensin system blockade. The dose of oral morphine should be 2.5–5 mg initially, and titrated up as needed and tolerated. Alternative opioids such as immediate-release oxycodone or low-dose fentanyl patches may also be useful. Prescription can be on a regular or as-required basis. It is usually well tolerated and common side effects can be anticipated and prophylactic treatment prescribed. Many patients require an anti-emetic, particularly during the first few days of treatment, and the majority require regular laxatives. The dose of morphine and its dose interval should be regularly reviewed and adjusted appropriately in the context of significant side effects, including oversedation. Older patients in particular are at risk of a deteriorating renal function, which can result in the poor clearance of opioids and potentially opioid toxicity. Some patients may incorrectly associate the initiation of morphine therapy with imminent death. It is important therefore, that the symptomatic benefits in the longer term are fully explained to the patient in order to avoid any unnecessary anxiety.

Benzodiazepines

To date, no studies have been reported assessing the use of benzodiazepines to alleviate dyspnoea in patients with HF. However, in practice, it appears that patients with advanced HF and refractory dyspnoea may benefit from them. Benzodiazepines may be particularly effective in patients where dyspnoea is accompanied by significant anxiety and distress. Possible regimes include sublingual lorazepam 0.5–1 mg as required, or subcutaneous midazolam 2.5–5 mg. As with opioids, short-acting benzodiazepines are preferred and the dose interval should be regularly reviewed. There is evidence that the clearance of benzodiazepines is reduced in patients with chronic HF, and this will be exacerbated by any deterioration in renal function [32]. Specific caution should also be exercised when prescribing benzodiazepines to older patients as this may increase the risk of falls [33]. One small study demonstrated that a nocturnal prescription of temazepam improved sleep patterns in patients with moderate to severe chronic HF, without any deterioration in oxygen saturations [34].

Non-pharmacological measures

Dyspnoea in patients with advanced HF may be improved by various simple, non-pharmacological measures. These may include upright positioning, the use of an electric fan, pacing and prioritizing various relaxation strategies. Patients can also learn specific breathing techniques, and indeed there is evidence that slowing the respiratory rate can reduce the symptoms of dyspnoea and improve both resting gas exchange and exercise tolerance in patients with HF [35].

Oedema

Oedema is a common clinical feature in patients with advanced and terminal heart failure [36], and can be particularly distressing during the later stages of the disease. Such oedema can lead to lower-limb discomfort, the breakdown of skin, blistering and infection and consequent fluid seepage from the lower limbs, and is a common reason for readmission to hospital. Thus, the optimum use of diuretics is of great importance (see below).

The early detection of oedema is key to its effective management, and the patient and family should be alerted to early signs of oedema and weight gain.

It is essential that the aetiology of worsening oedema is identified. It may be that it simply reflects the heart failure, but other factors such as poor compliance with fluid restriction or medical therapy should also be considered. Other causes of lower-limb swelling, such renal insufficiency, hepatic insufficiency, cellulitis and deep-vein thrombosis, should be kept in mind.

Generally, intravenous diuretics are required and currently in most cases this necessitates admission to hospital. Bolus doses of intravenous loop diuretics (e.g. furosemide) may be supplemented with oral thiazides such as bendrofluazide or metolazone. Spironolactone may also reduce oedema, although the patient's potassium levels must be carefully monitored. In the context of renal insufficiency diuresis may be improved by the addition of 'renal-dose' dopamine, although convincing evidence for this is lacking. Fluid restriction to 1.5 l per day is worth considering to lessen the oedema, but this measure should be short term and a pragmatic approach adopted. Daily weight measurements to assess the reduction in peripheral oedema are useful, and a weight loss of no more than 0.5–1 kg per day will reduce the likelihood of hypovolaemia and its attendant risks. In addition, any illness leading to hypovolaemia and dehydration may also worsen the situation.

A close monitoring of renal function is indicated as long as intravenous diuretics are felt to be appropriate. Physical measures such as a period of bed rest and lower-limb elevation often contribute significantly to reducing the oedema.

Skin care is important in patients with advanced HF and peripheral oedema. Patients often complain of dry and itchy skin, and so the prescription of an aqueous moisturizer is useful. Pressure-relieving mattresses and heel protectors are important adjuncts for bed-bound patients. Dry skin, particularly if oedematous, may provide a portal of entry for infection and so cellulitis in these patients is common. This should be promptly treated, usually with intravenous antibiotics, as patients with advanced heart failure will have little reserve in the context of septicaemia.

Fatigue

Fatigue is a major manifestation of advanced HF. In a recent study of symptoms during the last six months of life in advanced HF patients, fatigue was reported by 69% of patients [20]. While fatigue may be secondary to heart failure *per se*, it can also be exacerbated by other factors that are common in advanced HF patients.

- Patients who have responded poorly to conventional medical management may experience refractory orthopnoea and recurrent paroxysmal dyspnoea, with an adverse effect on sleep patterns. Simple interventions such as raising the patient's feet in the bed to prevent slipping down may be helpful.

- Cheyne–Stokes respiration and periodic breathing secondary to augmented chemosensitivity may also result in disrupted sleep patterns. Studies have suggested that hyperoxia, dihydrocodeine or temazepam may ameliorate this [34, 37]. Nocturnal apnoea may also be improved by noninvasive ventilation.

- Nutritional intake is frequently inadequate in patients with advanced HF, and this may also contribute to fatigue [38].

- Fatigue may be secondary to beta-blockade, and a dose reduction or withdrawal of beta-blockade may appropriate, particularly in terminal HF.

- Other potentially reversible comorbidities to consider are anaemia, perhaps secondary to chronic disease or to antiplatelet or anticoagulant therapy, hypo-kalaemia secondary to diuretic therapy, hypothyroidism and depression, each of which is more common in older patients with advanced HF (see Chapter 8).

Pain

Pain in advanced HF is common, as evidenced by the SUPPORT study in which 43% of patients reported significant pain, and only 10% being satisfied with the level of analgesia received. The pain is multifactorial; it may be secondary to an acute coronary syndrome, refractory angina or to gastrointestinal congestion, gross oedema, gout or immobility. Other comorbidities may also contribute, including diabetic neuropathy and, particularly in older patients, osteoarthritis. In the management of pain in these patients the World Health organization (WHO) analgesic ladder can be employed [40]. However, non-steroidal anti-inflammatory drugs should be avoided due to their propensity to cause fluid retention and adversely affect renal function. Opioids should be commenced at small doses and titrated cautiously. Angina refractory to conventional treatment may respond to opioids or may require other measures such as an implantable spinal cord stimulator or enhanced external pneumatic counterpulsation. Neuropathic pain may be improved by anticonvulsant drugs such as gabapentin, although unfortunately this causes fluid retention in up to 10% of patients and the dose must be reduced if the patient has renal impairment. Tricyclic antidepressants such as amitriptyline should be avoided due to the risk of inducing an arrhythmia.

Difficult, refractory pain, for example from limb ischaemia, may require specialist palliative medicine input and the use of alternative analgesics such as ketamine or methadone.

14.5 Home and hospital care

Although hospitalization will be necessary from time to time to allow more intensive therapy, it is often difficult to judge when hospital admission is necessary. A balance must be struck between the risks of inappropriately delaying hospitalization against the psychological and other benefits of care at home, and the decision whether or not to hospitalize depends on many factors (see Tables 14.2 and 14.3). Further developments are needed to take the end-of-life care of patients with HF to a level where home management can be delivered at an equivalent standard to hospice care right up until the time of death. Some centres do adopt a 'hospital at home'

Table 14.2 Categories of problems which suggest that hospitalization might be medically beneficial.

- No satisfactory explanation for current deterioration.
- The prospect of being able to effectively treat the cause of the patient's deterioration which cannot be accurately diagnosed or treated at home, for example acute cardiac pain.
- The need for therapy which cannot be delivered or monitored in the community.
- Patient/carer distress and/or inability of carer to cope at home.

Table 14.3 Specific indications for hospitalization.

- Need for intravenous therapy
- Pulmonary oedema with distress
- Refractory oedema despite high-dose oral therapy
- Fluid leakage from lower limbs
- Symptomatic postural hypotension
- Symptomatic arrhythmia
- Refractory pain
- Anaemia requiring blood transfusion

approach for episodes of decompensation and for terminal care, with infusions of diuretics (intravenously or subcutaneously) given at home, although currently the infrastructure to achieve this is not often in place (see below and Chapter 13).

14.6   Withdrawal of conventional drugs

When a patient is deemed to have terminal heart failure, it is inappropriate to continue to prescribe the majority of routine medications. Hence, a balance must be established between drugs that are of benefit in terms of survival, and those of which the principal benefit is the alleviation of symptoms (see Table 14.1).

This means that most conventional therapies for heart failure (ACE inhibitors, angiotensin II receptor blockers, aldosterone and beta-blockers) should usually be discontinued and their symptom-relieving properties replaced by appropriate palliative care protocols (see below). An added reason for discontinuing these drugs is that their mechanism of action includes a hypotensive effect, and in many of these patients the blood pressure will already be low. In addition, the patients will be more prone to hypovolaemia because of a reduced fluid intake. The two groups of agents in the conventional category which could still be of help in the terminal phase are diuretics and digoxin. Diuretics in particular may continue to assist in relieving distressing oedema and preventing pulmonary oedema with its attendant dyspnoea. However, in patients with terminal heart failure the aggressive management of oedema is inappropriate, intravenous access is often difficult, impractical or deemed undesirable, and the same is true for oral medication. In these circumstances the administration of furosemide by the subcutaneous route may be a valid alternative [41, 42].

Digoxin, provided that the dose is monitored closely, may be symptomatically beneficial by reducing heart rate and dyspnoea without adversely affecting the blood pressure [15].

14.7   The palliative care needs of heart failure patients

Recognition of the physical and mental distress of patients with terminal heart failure effectively began a little over 10 years ago, triggered by two reports which detailed the poorly controlled cardiac and noncardiac symptoms of heart failure patients during the final stages of their illness [43,44]. In the subsequent 10 years, notably in the US and UK, individual cardiologists, GPs and palliative care teams have collaborated to develop local – and, in the UK – national strategies to address these and related problems. These strategies [5, 45] are based largely on the Gold Standard Framework (GSF) [3] and the Liverpool Care Pathway for the Dying Patient (LCP) [2]. These reports and guidelines highlight the palliative care needs of patients with heart failure and detail how they can be resolved.

Patients with heart failure:

- Have a worse prognosis than most patients with other progressive diseases.

- Unlike with many other life-limiting diseases, symptoms can impose restrictions on daily activities from an early stage of the disease, which then become increasingly resistant to conventional treatment as it progresses.

- Patients commonly have multiple comorbidities that sometimes dominate the clinical picture but are often either ignored or treated inadequately (see Chapter 8).

- The quality of life is worse than that of virtually all other chronic life-limiting conditions.

There are other, generic, problems often faced by heart failure patients:

- A lack of communication between patients and their professional carers, as a result of which they are ill-informed about their condition and management plans.

- Care is fragmented and poorly coordinated.

- There is often a failure by professionals to identify (or to acknowledge) when a patient is terminally ill, and this leads to inappropriately active treatment.

Three general comments are pertinent to addressing the patients' needs:

- Most of the palliative care needs of patients with heart failure respond to the same treatments and management strategies as those of patients with other progressive diseases.

- In broad terms, the same palliative care treatments and management strategies are appropriate for older and younger heart failure patients. However, as noted above, there are additional problems largely confined to older patients, which may complicate the implementation of these strategies.

- The different components of palliative and supportive care strategies which are appropriate for heart failure patients, and the timing of their introduction, is based on an understanding of patients' changing needs as their condition deteriorates.

14.8 Palliative care strategies for heart failure

In the light of the inadequacies of conventional treatment to address patients' needs, as noted above, each of the main palliative care strategies is relevant to patients with heart failure:

- Improving communication with them and between health care professionals.

- Treatment for poorly controlled symptoms.

- Advanced care planning and providing support in the community.

- The provision of optimum end-of-life care.

The latter three strategies are particularly needed when the patient is identified as having reached the stage of advanced heart failure.

The palliative care needs of 90% of heart failure patients can be managed by using what the National Institute for Health and Clinical Excellence (NICE) defines as basic palliative care [46] – skills which can be acquired by any doctors or nurses working with these patients. The direct involvement of palliative care teams in patient management is therefore only needed occasionally.

The NICE definition of 'general (basic) palliative care'

- Assessment of patient and carer need for support.

- Open and sensitive communication.

- Coordination of services (throughout 24 h and across boundaries).

- Basic level of symptom control.

- Psychological, social, spiritual and practical support.

- Appropriate referral for specialist palliative care.

Based on Ref. [46].

14.9 Timing the introduction of different palliative care strategies

The only way to identify the physical and psychosocial needs of individual patients is by regularly reviewing and discussing with them their unresolved personal concerns, whether they be physical, psychological, 'spiritual' or social.

Communication

Good communication is in many ways as important to the patients' well-being as other aspects of their management, and is the one component of palliative care which should be routinely introduced from the time of diagnosis.

The effectiveness of communication with patients is entirely dependent on their comprehension of, and active involvement in, the topics under discussion; whether it is to discuss their condition, its treatment or other important issues, or to obtain informed permission for treatment. This is, in the UK, dependent on the patient's mental capacity as defined by the Mental Capacity Act 2005 in England and Wales and in the Adults with Incapacity Act 2000 in Scotland [47]. The discussion of issues such as cardiopulmonary resuscitation or advance decisions (see below) are specific examples where mental capacity is needed and is particularly relevant to older patients in whom cognitive impairment is common.

A recurring complaint from heart failure patients and/or their carers is that they are poorly informed about their condition and its management, that they are excluded from decision making about their care, and that staff do not allow them time to talk about their personal concerns. Unless these issues are addressed, the patients and their carers become frustrated, angry and anxious, and their quality of life deteriorates [48, 49].

Not surprisingly therefore, good communication is one of the central tenets of palliative care and involves much more than telling patients what is wrong and the proposed treatment:

- It is based on specific communication skills described as active listening, the skills to empathetically break bad news to them, and therapeutic dialogue.

- The necessary expertise has to be learned, just as are any other clinical skills [50, 51].

- Many patients and their carers also appreciate having written information about their diagnosis, prognosis and management.

- Some of the issues which should be discussed with patients and their carers are generic, others are mainly pertinent to those with heart failure.

Communication and generic issues

Advance decisions

An advance decision ('living will'),

- Is a written statement made by a person when they are competent (i.e. have the necessary mental capacity), detailing the circumstances under which they would not wish to receive life-prolonging treatment should they later become unable to express their wishes.

- It is a legally binding document [47].

In practical terms it would be ideal if all patients signed an advance decision, and an appropriate occasion should therefore be sought to discuss it. This could avoid the need to raise difficult issues such as cardiopulmonary resuscitation and the deactivation of implantable cardioverter defibrillators at the end of the patient's life.

Psychosocial, spiritual and financial issues

A range of topics come under this heading which are largely ignored by many clinicians. However, if they are not adequately addressed they can have a worse impact on the well-being of patients and carers than their physical symptoms and limitations.

Psychological issues

- Fear, anger, depression and denial are generic coping strategies of people with life-threatening diseases.

- Loss of physical independence and a feeling of being a burden are common issues.

- These problems may lead to stress within families and with friends.

- Most health care professionals (HCPs) have little experience of addressing these difficult issues.

- The necessary skills can be acquired by HCPs caring for heart failure patients through locally organized training programmes.

Social and financial needs

- Many patients with advanced heart failure are housebound and, especially those who are older, socially isolated.

- Patients with progressive diseases are frequently concerned about their ability to cope financially and about the impact that this has on their families [52, 53].

- A key health care worker should be identified to coordinate the implementation of appropriate financial and social support.

Spiritual needs

'Spiritual' is a much misunderstood word; its importance to patients with a limited prognosis is consistently overlooked.

- It is not synonymous with religious belief.

- It encompasses any of our experiences or emotions which give comfort, pleasure and meaning to life, for example family and friends or the appreciation of beauty in any of its forms.

- The prospect of losing family, friends or sources of comfort, or the inability to find satisfactory answers to a range of personal questions may be more distressing to the patient and carers than intractable physical symptoms [54].

For many centuries the heart has been seen as the seat of the soul. It has a special place, more than a pump which sustains life. Even the word 'failure' has undertones of blame and falling short. Spiritual pain encompasses loss, guilt and anxiety. Above all, it relates to meaning and purpose. At a superficial level spiritual pain is caused by less of a role as husband, lover and breadwinner or as a mother, friend or carer of others. Deeper spiritual pain relates to existential issues. 'Why me, what have I done?' Support is first of all to accept the above aims as real, then to enable the patient to explore what has helped at times of distress in the past. The preferred professional attitude is best described as not seeking a neat answer, or indeed regarding spiritual suffering as a problem to be solved. Helping to cope with spiritual pain may require just a presence.

14.10 Cardiological issues

Sudden cardiac death

Between 40–50% of patients with heart failure die suddenly and unexpectedly, usually because of an arrhythmia or an acute coronary ischaemic event. This is most likely to occur during the earlier stages of heart failure [55]. The subject should therefore be broached early in the course of the disease so that patients and carers are prepared for this eventuality.

Cardiopulmonary resuscitation (CPR) and do not attempt resuscitation (DNAR) orders

Three points are particularly relevant to patients with advanced heart failure, bearing in mind that it is widely believed that CPR will be unsuccessful in this situation, that even in those in whom it is initially successful survival to discharge is unlikely, and that age is an independent risk factor for unsuccessful CPR.

- Doctors have a duty to act in the best interests of the patient; that is, they should offer treatment which improves symptoms, prognosis and/or quality of life.

- There is no legal requirement to offer a treatment which is unlikely to be effective, or which is likely to cause harm.

- Issues relating to CPR should always be discussed with patients or, if this would be inappropriate, with their carers. It should always be discussed with those who have indicated that they wish to be involved in decisions about their care.

- DNAR orders should always be documented to avoid inappropriate CPR attempts.

Deactivation of implantable cardioverter defibrillators (ICDs)

An ICD in effect automatically initiates CPR with the objective of restoring sinus rhythm. Logically, if CPR is judged to be inappropriate, then a patient's ICD should be deactivated.

- If still functioning at the time of death, the device will continue to deliver shocks to the patient. This may be visible to family or friends who are present, and is likely to cause them distress.

- Deactivation of the device is a simple, brief and painless procedure undertaken by cardiology department technicians.

- Discussion about a possible future recommendation for this to be done should be initiated at the time of implantation; failing this, it should be programmed into the patient's advance care plan (see below).

- A detailed discussion of this topic is provided by the British Heart Foundation [56].

14.11   The management implications of advanced heart failure

Usually, when a person's health deteriorates, so too does their quality of life (QOL). Most doctors are used to treating patients to relieve symptoms and/or prolong life, and it is tacitly assumed that an improvement in QOL will follow; they have little first-hand experience of treatment, the primary purpose of which is to improve the QOL. However, when faced with a patient whose symptoms are resistant to conventional treatment, whose QOL is poor and who will clearly continue to deteriorate, it is illogical to persevere exclusively with a failing strategy when there is a better alternative. This is the situation with patients who have advanced heart failure.

Advanced heart failure, as defined above, is in practice identified with hindsight. But nevertheless it represents a watershed in the patient's management.

The reality of advanced heart failure:

- By definition, conventional treatment will not result in additional relief of the classical symptoms.

- The need for hospitalization, triggered by worsening heart failure and its complications, medication-related problems or a comorbidity becomes more common.

- Patients are increasingly housebound and, especially those who are older and/or female, socially isolated.

Throughout this stage palliative care should be incrementally introduced as appropriate, complementing not replacing conventional treatment.

Some rules of thumb for when to consider palliative care

- A request from a patient or their family for palliative care warrants serious consideration. It implies that they have taken the trouble to investigate palliative care themselves, and that they may already have symptoms needing attention.

Such requests are usually appropriate. Even if the patient's current problems are under control, those living in the UK should be placed on the primary care palliative care register and should also be registered under the Gold Standards Framework which provides a comprehensive method of keeping such patients under review as their condition deteriorates (see below).

- Health professionals involved in the management of patients with heart failure should ask themselves, when seeing a patient, 'Would I be surprised if this patient died within one year'. If the answer is 'no' – which is clearly the case in patients with advanced heart failure (the annual mortality being 30–50%) – then their palliative care needs should be assessed.

- If the patient has had at least one admission to hospital for heart failure.

14.12   Control of symptoms using mostly generic treatments

The control of both cardiac and noncardiac symptoms is demonstrably poor [43, 57], and is increasingly so as patients deteriorate. Detailed accounts of generic symptom control protocols are provided in published and local palliative care guidelines, some of which are discussed above ('Management of specific symptoms'), while conventional medications used to treat heart failure are detailed in Table 14.1.

Two principles of management should be applied before introducing palliative care measures for symptom control:

- Ensuring that the patient is receiving the optimum conventional treatment for heart failure (see Chapter 6) – and for angina when needed.

- The identification of any reversible cause for cardiac and noncardiac symptoms; for example, an iatrogenic cause for gastrointestinal symptoms.

14.13   Support in the community: the gold standard framework (GSF) and advanced care planning (ACP)

For 95% of the time, patients with heart failure are managed in the community by their local health care team – which ideally will include a specialist heart failure nurse.

The GSF [3] is widely used in the UK and is a nationally recommended [51] generic programme of strategies, tasks and enabling tools designed to help primary care teams to improve the organization and quality of care for patients during the last 12 months of life, whether at home, in community hospitals or in care homes. The GSF is based on three principles:

- The identification of patients in need of palliative/supportive care towards the end of life.

- Assessing patients' symptoms, preferences and any other issues important to them.

- Planning care which prioritizes patients' needs and preferences. This includes helping people to live and to die where they choose; increasingly, the choice is to die at home [5].

The objectives of an ACP strategy are to provide:

- Better collaboration between primary and secondary health care teams.

- Improved communication between individuals, teams, patients and carers to increase patient involvement in decision making and to reduce the chances of receiving confusing or conflicting advice.

- The introduction of a strategy to ensure integrated 24 h care when needed.

Patients with advanced heart failure are often hospitalized because of worsening or new symptoms (see below). This may be clinically appropriate, but in other cases it

Table 14.4 Factors suggesting that hospitalization is not appropriate.

- The patient does not wish to be hospitalized
- Recent hospitalization or outpatient clinic visits to treat deteriorating cardiac function produced neither objective nor subjective improvement
- The patient is unsuitable, or does not wish to be considered for further active treatment

may be unnecessary or contrary to their wishes (Table 14.4); thus, the ACP component of the GSF is designed to avoid unnecessary or unwanted hospitalization by encouraging appropriate care and support in the community for patient and carers (see also Chapter 12).

Despite these scenarios, if the patient is thought to be terminally ill (see below) and/or has expressed a wish, either verbally or as an advance decision to remain at home, then moving them to hospital is rarely justified. Currently, although two-thirds of patients would prefer to die at home, less than half of this number do so.

14.14 Terminal heart failure: identifying the dying patient and providing end-of-life care

As noted above, this term is applied to patients who are thought likely to die within the next few days. There may have been a gradual deterioration in health, or the terminal stage may have been triggered by an acute irreversible event such as an acute coronary syndrome.

Although there are no diagnostic criteria of terminal heart failure, there are a number of clinical pointers (some generic and some cardiological) which, when several occur in combination, strongly suggest that this stage may have been reached (Table 14.5).

For a number of reasons, doctors often fail to recognize or are reluctant to accept that this is the case. In some situations there are valid reasons for this reluctance:

- The need to ensure, as noted above, that the current situation is irreversible.

- Varying the combination and dosages of conventional heart failure medications may temporarily relieve breathlessness, oedema or renal dysfunction.

The reluctance to initiate an appropriate end-of-life care strategy is also partly based on a misunderstanding of the optimum management of the dying process. It is a gradual merging of active, palliative and terminal care strategies; it is not a sudden change in direction, nor does it constitute euthanasia.

Table 14.5 Cardiological and generic indicators of terminal heart failure.

Generic pointers:
    Unable to take oral medication or fluids
    Increasingly withdrawn and unresponsive
    Weak/exhausted
    Bed-bound
    Delirium

Heart failure-related pointers:
    Identified as having refractory symptoms
    Recent hospitalization or outpatient visits without benefit.
    No reversible cause for current deterioration
    NYHA class IV
    Life-threatening comorbidity

Be that as it may, failure to consider that patients who fulfil the 'terminally ill criteria' may die in the near future can result in them having inappropriate treatment [44]:

- Poor symptom control.

- Inappropriate interventions, for example tube feeding or artificial ventilation in the last 48 h of life.

- A lack of spiritual or religious support for them and their carers.

- Their treatment preferences being ignored.

When the medical team members agree that the terminal stage has been reached, the patient and their carers should be advised of the situation and that, with their agreement, care should now be based on the LCP [2] or a comparable end-of-life care pathway. It is now generally agreed that simply providing symptom relief (e.g. for the common terminal symptoms) is inadequate to address the complexities of optimally managing the terminally ill.

The LCP ensures:

- Clear, agreed, clinical decisions

- Teamwork

- Effective communication with colleagues, patients and carers

- Symptomatic relief of physical and other forms of distress

- Regular checks on the patient and family

Table 14.6　Summary of treatment for common generic symptoms in the terminally ill.[a]

Respiratory tract secretions:
　　Positional change may help
　　Antimuscarinic drugs, for example hyoscine hydrobromide (or -n-butylbromide) or
　　　glycopyrronium: these should be given as soon as symptoms occur
　　Suction may be needed

Nausea and vomiting:
　　Treat specifically any identified underlying pathology
　　Medications include cyclizine, metoclopramine, antimuscarinics, levomepromazine

Restlessness and confusion:
　　Identify and treat specific precipitant for example metabolic upset, drug toxicity
　　A benzodiazepine (e.g. midazolam)
　　For resistant symptoms, haloperidol or levomepromazine

[a]Medicines should only be prescribed on advice given in local or published guidelines. Based on data from Ref. [58].

- Discontinuation of non-essential drugs (see Table 14.1)

- Interventional procedures and regular monitoring are discontinued

- Attention to details.

Details of symptom control are provided in local palliative care programmes and in national and other published guidelines. A summary of some of the treatments for the more common symptoms of the terminally ill is provided in Table 14.6.

References

1. World Health Organization (2007) Palliative Care. http://www.who.int/cancer/palliative/en/ (last accessed 19 April 2007).
2. Liverpool Care. Pathway for the Care of the Dying. www.lcp-mariecurie.org.uk.
3. The Gold Standard Framework website: http://www.goldstandardsframework.nhs.uk/.
4. NHS Modernisation Agency Coronary Heart Disease Collaborative (2004) *Supportive and Palliative Care for Advanced Heart Failure*, Department of Health, London.
5. Scottish Partnership for Palliative Care (2008) *Living and Dying with Advanced Heart Failure: A Palliative Care Approach*. Scottish Partnership for Palliative Care, Edinburgh.
6. Adams, K.F. Jr and Zannad, F. (1998) Clinical definition and epidemiology of advanced heart failure. *American Heart Journal*, **135** (6 Pt 2 Su), S204–S215.
7. The SOLVD Investigators (1991) Effect of enalapril on survival in patients with reduced left ventricular ejection fractions and congestive heart failure. *New England Journal of Medicine*, **325** (5), 293–302.

8. Pfeffer, M.A., McMurray, J.J., Velazquez, E.J. *et al.* (2003) Valsartan, captopril, or both in myocardial infarction complicated by heart failure, left ventricular dysfunction, or both. *New England Journal of Medicine*, **349** (20), 1893–1906.

9. Pfeffer, M.A., Swedberg, K., Granger, C.B. *et al.* (2003) Effects of candesartan on mortality and morbidity in patients with chronic heart failure: the CHARM-Overall programme. *Lancet*, **362** (9386), 759–766.

10. Pitt, B., Zannad, F., Remme, W.J. *et al.* (1999) The effect of spironolactone on morbidity and mortality in patients with severe heart failure. Randomized Aldactone Evaluation Study Investigators. *New England Journal of Medicine*, **341** (10), 709–717.

11. Tendera, M. and Ochala, A. (2001) Overview of the results of recent beta blocker trials. *Current Opinion in Cardiology*, **16** (3), 180–185.

12. Masoudi, F.A., Wolfe, P., Havranek, E.P. *et al.* (2005) Aspirin use in older patients with heart failure and coronary artery disease: national prescription patterns and relationship with outcomes. *Journal of the American College of Cardiology*, **46** (6), 955–962.

13. Sacks, F.M., Pfeffer, M.A., Moye, L.A. *et al.* (1996) The effect of pravastatin on coronary events after myocardial infarction in patients with average cholesterol levels. Cholesterol and Recurrent Events Trial investigators. *New England Journal of Medicine*, **335** (14), 1001–1009.

14. Faris, R., Flather, M.D., Purcell, H. *et al.* (2006) Diuretics for heart failure. *Cochrane Database of Systematic Reviews* 1, CD003838.

15. The Digitalis Investigation Group (1997) The effect of digoxin on mortality and morbidity in patients with heart failure. *New England Journal of Medicine*, **336** (8), 525–533.

16. Pappone, C. and Santinelli, V. (2004) The who, what, why, and how-to guide for circumferential pulmonary vein ablation. *Journal of Cardiovascular Electrophysiology*, **15** (10), 1226–1230.

17. Cleland, J.G., Daubert, J.C., Erdmann, E. *et al.* (2005) The effect of cardiac resynchronization on morbidity and mortality in heart failure. *New England Journal of Medicine*, **352** (15), 1539–1549.

18. Bristow, M.R., Feldman, A.M. and Saxon, L.A. (2000) Heart failure management using implantable devices for ventricular resynchronization: Comparison of Medical Therapy, Pacing, and Defibrillation in Chronic Heart Failure (COMPANION) trial. COMPANION Steering Committee and COMPANION Clinical Investigators. *Journal of Cardiac Failure*, **6** (3), 276–285.

19. Mueller, P.S., Jenkins, S.M., Bramstedt, K.A. *et al.* (2008) Deactivating implanted cardiac devices in terminally ill patients: practices and attitudes. *Pacing and Clinical Electrophysiology*, **31** (5), 560–568.

20. Nordgren, L. and Sorensen, S. (2003) Symptoms experienced in the last six months of life in patients with end-stage heart failure. *European Journal of Cardiovascular Nursing*, **2** (3), 213–217.

21. Johnson, M.J. (2007) Management of end stage cardiac failure. *Postgraduate Medical Journal*, **83** (980), 395–401.

22. Moore, D.P., Weston, A.R., Hughes, J.M. *et al.* (1992) Effects of increased inspired oxygen concentrations on exercise performance in chronic heart failure. *Lancet,* **339** (8797), 850–853.

23. Restrick, L.J., Davies, S.W., Noone, L. *et al.* (1992) Ambulatory oxygen in chronic heart failure. *Lancet,* **340** (8829), 1192–1193.

24. Russell, S.D., Koshkarian, G.M., Medinger, A.E. *et al.* (1999) Lack of effect of increased inspired oxygen concentrations on maximal exercise capacity or ventilation in stable heart failure. *American Journal of Cardiology,* **84** (12), 1412–1416.

25. Booth, S., Wade, R., Johnson, M. *et al.* (2004) The use of oxygen in the palliation of breathlessness. A report of the expert working group of the Scientific Committee of the Association of Palliative Medicine. *Respiratory Medicine,* **98** (1), 66–77.

26. Lorenz, K.A., Lynn, J., Dy, S.M. *et al.* (2008) Evidence for improving palliative care at the end of life: a systematic review. *Annals of Internal Medicine,* **148** (2), 147–159.

27. Clark, A.L. and McDonagh, T. (1997) The origin of symptoms in chronic heart failure. *Heart,* **78** (5), 429–430.

28. Chua, T.P., Harrington, D., Ponikowski, P. *et al.* (1997) Effects of dihydrocodeine on chemosensitivity and exercise tolerance in patients with chronic heart failure. *Journal of the American College of Cardiology,* **29** (1), 147–152.

29. Johnson, M.J., McDonagh, T.A., Harkness, A. *et al.* (2002) Morphine for the relief of breathlessness in patients with chronic heart failure – a pilot study. *European Journal of Heart Failure,* **4** (6), 753–756.

30. Farncombe, M. and Chater, S. (1993) Case studies outlining use of nebulized morphine for patients with end-stage chronic lung and cardiac disease. *Journal of Pain and Symptom Management,* **8** (4), 221–225.

31. Williams, S.G., Wright, D.J., Marshall, P. *et al.* (2003) Safety and potential benefits of low dose diamorphine during exercise in patients with chronic heart failure. *Heart,* **89** (9), 1085–1086.

32. Patel, I.H., Soni, P.P., Fukuda, E.K. *et al.* (1990) The pharmacokinetics of midazolam in patients with congestive heart failure. *British Journal of Clinical Pharmacology,* **29** (5), 565–569.

33. Gales, B.J. and Menard, S.M. (1995) Relationship between the administration of selected medications and falls in hospitalized elderly patients. *Annals of Pharmacotherapy,* **29** (4), 354–358.

34. Biberdorf, D.J., Steens, R., Millar, T.W. *et al.* (1993) Benzodiazepines in congestive heart failure. *Sleep,* **16** (6), 529–538.

35. Bernardi, L., Spadacini, G., Bellwon, J. *et al.* (1998) Effect of breathing rate on oxygen saturation and exercise performance in chronic heart failure. *Lancet,* **351** (9112), 1308–1311.

36. Nordgren, L. and Sorensen, S. (2003) Symptoms experienced in the last six months of life in patients with end-stage heart failure. *European Journal of Cardiovascular Nursing,* **2** (3), 213–217.

37. Ponikowski, P., Anker, S.D., Chua, T.P. *et al.* (1999) Oscillatory breathing patterns during wakefulness in patients with chronic heart failure: clinical implications and role of augmented peripheral chemosensitivity. *Circulation*, **100** (24), 2418–2424.

38. Catapano, G., Pedone, C., Nunziata, E. *et al.* (2008) Nutrient intake and serum cytokine pattern in elderly people with heart failure. *European Journal of Heart Failure*, **10** (4), 428–434.

39. Levenson, J.W., McCarthy, E.P., Lynn, J. *et al.* (2000) The last six months of life for patients with congestive heart failure. *Journal of the American Geriatric Society*, **48** (5 Suppl), S101–S109.

40. World Health Organization (1996) *Cancer Pain Relief*, 2nd edition, World Health Organization, Geneva.

41. Verma, A.K., da Silva, J.H. and Kuhl, D.R. (2004) Diuretic effects of subcutaneous furosemide in human volunteers: a randomized pilot study. *Annals of Pharmacotherapy*, **38** (4), 544–549.

42. Goenaga, M.A., Millet, M., Sanchez, E. *et al.* (2004) Subcutaneous furosemide. *Annals of Pharmacotherapy*, **38** (10), 1751.

43. McCarthy, M., Lay, M. and Addington-Hall, J. (1996) Dying from heart disease. *Journal of the Royal College Physician of London*, **30**, 325–328.

44. Lynne, J., Teno, J.M., Phillips, R.S. *et al.* for the SUPPORT Group Members (1997) Perceptions by family members of the dying experience of older and seriously ill patients. *Annals of Internal Medicine*, **126** (2), 97–106.

45. Coronary Heart Disease Collaborative: Supportive and palliative care for advanced heart failure. www.modern.nhs.uk/chd.

46. National Institute for Clinical Excellence (NICE) (2004) *Improving Supportive and Palliative Care for Adults with Cancer*. Royal College of Physicians, London. Available at www.nice.org.uk.

47. British Medical Association (2007) Advance decisions and proxy decision-making in medical treatment and research, Guidance from the BMA's medical Ethics Department. British Medical Association, London.

48. McCarthy, M. and Addington-Hall, J. (1997) Communication and choice in dying from heart disease. *Journal of the Royal Society of Medicine*, **90**, 128–131.

49. Boyd, K.J., Murray, S.A., Kendall, M. *et al.* (2004) Living with advanced heart failure: a prospective, community based study of patients and their carers. *European Journal of Heart Failure*, **6** (5), 585–591.

50. Kaye, P. (1996) *Breaking Bad News: A Ten Step Approach*, EPL Publications, 41 Park Avenue North, Northampton, NN3 2HT.

51. NHS End of Life Care Programme (2007) Department of Health, London. Available at www.endoflifecare.nhs.uk.

52. Kuter, J., Steiner, J., Corbett, K. *et al.* (1999) Information needs in terminal illness. *Social Science and Medicine*, **48**, 1341–1352.

53. Thomas, C. and Morris, S. (2001) *What are the Psychosocial Needs of Cancer Patients and their Main Carer?* Institute of Health Research, Lancaster University.

54. Scottish Partnership for Palliative Care (2006) *Joined Up Thinking - Joined Up Care.* Scottish Partnership for Palliative Care, Edinburgh.

55. MERIT-HF study Group (1999) Effect of metoprolol CR/XL in chronic heart failure: Metoprolol CR/XL Randomised Intervention Trial in Congestive Cardiac Failure (MERIT-HF). *Lancet*, **353**, 2001–2007.

56. British Heart Foundation (2007) Implantable cardioverter defibrillators in patients who are reaching the end of life A discussion document for health professionals. www.bhf.org. uk/publications.

57. Anderson, H., Ward, C. and Eardley, A. (2001) The concerns of patients under palliative care and a heart failure clinic are not being met. *Palliative Medicine*, **15** (4), 279–286.

58. Glare, P., Dickman, A. and Goodman, M. (2003) Symptom control in care of the dying, in *Care of the Dying: A Pathway to Excellence* (eds J. Ellershawe and S. Wilkinson), Oxford University Press, pp. 42–61.

Index

Note: page numbers in *italics* refer to figures and tables

A Practical Guide to Heart Failure in Older People, Edited by C Ward and M D Witham
© 2009 John Wiley & Sons, Ltd